The Effective Management of Ovarian Cancer

The Effective Management of Ovarian Cancer

Edited by

Professor Allan B MacLean MD FRCOG
Professor and Head of Department of Obstetrics and Gynaecology,
Royal Free and University College Medical School, London, UK

Dr Martin Gore PhD FRCP
Consultant Cancer Physician, The Royal Marsden Hospital, London, UK

Professor Andrew Miles MSc MPhil PhD
UEL Professor of Health Services Research and UK Key Advances Series Organiser
at St Bartholomew's Hospital, London, UK

UEL University Centre for
Health Services Research

AESCULAPIUS MEDICAL PRESS
LONDON SAN FRANCISCO SYDNEY

THE ROYAL COLLEGE
OF OBSTETRICIANS
AND GYNAECOLOGISTS

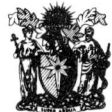

Published by

Aesculapius Medical Press (London, San Francisco, Sydney)
UEL University Centre for Health Services Research
St Bartholomew's Hospital
London EC1A 7BE

British Library Cataloguing in Publication Data

A catalogue record for this book is available from the British Library

ISBN 1 903044 02 2

While the advice and information in this book are believed to be true and accurate at the
time of going to press, neither the authors nor the publishers nor the collaborating
institutions can accept any legal responsibility or liability for any errors or omissions that
may be made. In particular (but without limiting the generality of the preceding
disclaimer) every effort has been made to check drug usages; however, it is possible that
errors have been missed. Furthermore, dosage schedules are constantly being revised and
new side-effects recognised. For these reasons, the reader is strongly urged to consult
the drug companies' printed instructions before administering any of the drugs
recommended in this book.

Further copies of this volume are available from:

Claudio Melchiorri
Research Dissemination Fellow
UEL Centre for Health Services Research
St Bartholomew's Hospital
London EC1 7BE

Fax: 0171 601 7085
E-mail: c.melchiorri@mds.qmw.ac.uk

Printed and bound in Great Britain by
Ashford Colour Press Ltd, Gosport, Hampshire

Contents

Contributors

Robbie Foy MFPHM MRCGP, Clinical Research Fellow, Scottish Programme for Clinical Effectiveness in Reproductive Health, Department of Obstetrics and Gynaecology, University of Edinburgh, Edinburgh, Scotland, UK

Martin Gore PhD FRCP, Consultant Cancer Physician, The Royal Marsden Hospital, London, UK

Ian Jacobs MD MRCOG, Professor/Consultant Gynaecological Oncologist, The Gynaecology Cancer Research Unit, St Bartholomew's Hospital, London, UK

Elizabeth Junor MD FRCP FRCR, Consultant Oncologist, Beatson Oncology Centre, Western Infirmary, Glasgow, Scotland, UK

Stan B Kaye BSc MD FRCP, Professor of Medical Oncology, CRC Department of Medical Oncology, University of Glasgow, and CRC Beatson Laboratories, Glasgow, Scotland, UK

Sean Kehoe MD DCH MRCOG, Senior Lecturer/Consultant Gynaecological Oncologist, Department of Gynaecological Oncology, City Hospital NHS Trust, Birmingham, UK

David Luesley MD FRCOG, Professor of Gynaecological Oncology, City Hospital NHS Trust, University of Birmingham, Birmingham, UK

Karen Maughan, Macmillan Nurse/Research Fellow, Gynaecological Oncology Centre, Queen Elizabeth Hospital, Gateshead, Tyne & Wear, UK

Chris Poole MA MB BChir FRCP, Macmillan Senior Lecturer, CRC Institute for Cancer Studies, University of Birmingham Medical School, Edgbaston, Birmingham, UK

Digumarti Raghunadharao MD DM(Med Onc), Associate Professor in Medical Oncology, Department of Medicine, Nizams Institute for Medical Sciences, Hyderbad, India

Wendy M N Reid MRCOG, Consultant Obstetrician & Gynaecologist, Department of Obstetrics & Gynaecology, Royal Free Hospital, London, UK

Adam N Rosenthal MB, Clinical Research Fellow, The Gynaecology Cancer Research Unit, St Bartholomew's Hospital, London, UK

Preface

It would seem self-evident that, in a disease such as ovarian cancer, where early-stage disease has a good prognosis and advanced disease is associated with a high mortality rate, screening strategies would provide a method of increasing survival. However, screening provides as many questions as answers because there are no randomised data showing a survival benefit. Research is still focused on which patients to screen, how often and by which method. In contrast, patients with a high familial risk of ovarian cancer are offered screening routinely because it is felt that a randomised clinical trial would be impossible in this patient group. Useful data will emerge from high-risk population-based studies such as the UKCCCR National Familial Ovarian Cancer Screening Study. Population-based randomised studies are in progress and they are of considerable importance.

Ovarian cancer provides a model for how cancer services should be provided to the community. It has been shown that survival is improved in patients who are managed by specialists working in teams and practising according to pre-set evidence-based guidelines. These teams can provide an important catalyst for the development of non-medical specialists such as clinical nurse specialists who can develop an important role in research and education for all health care professionals.

Surgery is an important modality of therapy and is curative for patients with early disease. It is also an adjunct to chemotherapy for patients with advanced disease. In patients with advanced disease, the amount of residual disease following surgery is a powerful prognostic indicator but there are still some controversies concerning the general role of surgery in relation to the biology of the disease. The timing of surgery remains an area requiring evaluation, in particular with regard to the strategy of interval debulking surgery during chemotherapy in patients with suboptimally debulked disease. Some randomised data support interval debulking surgery but confirmation is required and more precise data are needed in order to evaluate subsets of patients who would benefit most from this approach.

One of the most important advances in the management of ovarian cancer in the late 1970s and 1980s was the development of platinum compounds and the 1990s have seen the introduction of the taxanes. The first taxane developed was paclitaxel and randomised data have shown that platinum-paclitaxel combinations are superior to standard therapy. Future trials will now build on this observation in addition to the development of novel approaches that are based on a better understanding of the mechanisms of drug resistance and the targeting of the molecular events known to be involved in the development and maintenance of malignancy.

In the current age, where doctors and health professionals are increasingly overwhelmed by clinical information, we have aimed to provide a fully current, fully referenced text which is as succinct as possible but as comprehensive as necessary. Consultants and training grades in gynaecological, clinical and medical oncology will find it of particular use as part of continuing medical education and specialist training, and we advance it explicitly as an excellent tool for these purposes. We anticipate, however, that the book will prove of not inconsiderable use to oncology nurses and pharmacists as a reference text and to commissioners of health services as the basis for discussion and negotiation of health contracts with their practising colleagues.

In conclusion, we thank SmithKline Beecham Pharmaceuticals and Bristol-Myers Squibb Oncology UK for the grant of educational sponsorship which helped organise a national symposium of the Royal College of Obstetricians & Gynaecologists, at which synopses of the constituent chapters of this book were presented.

Allan B MacLean MD FRCOG
Martin Gore PhD FRCP
Andrew Miles MSc MPhil PhD

Chapter 1

Screening for pre-clinical ovarian cancer: progress and cost-effectiveness

Adam N Rosenthal and Ian J Jacobs

Introduction

Ovarian cancer is the commonest gynaecological malignancy in England and Wales and also has the highest case fatality rate of any gynaecological malignancy. Each year over 5,000 new cases are reported (OPCS 1994) and the current five-year survival rate is approximately 30-40 per cent (Nguyen *et al.* 1993). This poor prognosis has been attributed to late presentation (over 75 per cent of cases having extra-ovarian spread (Nguyen *et al.* 1993)). However, the five-year survival of patients presenting with disease limited to the pelvis is more favourable (over 90 per cent in stage Ia (Nguyen *et al.* 1993)), suggesting that detection of disease at an earlier stage may reduce mortality. Even if screening fails to detect stage I disease, evidence (van der Burg *et al.* 1995) suggests that optimal cytoreductive surgery may improve survival, implying that earlier detection of late-stage disease (i.e. stage IIIa or b, rather than IIIc) might improve prognosis.

It remains unclear as to whether the biology and natural history of ovarian cancer are amenable to screening. Evidence for a pre-malignant ovarian lesion is currently tenuous and little is known about the rate at which ovarian cancers grow and metastasise. The practical implications of these gaps in our knowledge are two-fold. First, we do not know how often to screen in order to avoid the occurrence of 'interval cancers' (cancers which present clinically between screens). Second, it is possible that current screening methods are detecting slow-growing tumours which may never cause problems, rather than the aggressive tumours which are responsible for most of the deaths from ovarian cancer.

Nevertheless, developments in tumour marker and ultrasound technology have provided us with tests which can detect a large majority of ovarian cancers before they cause symptoms. There is now sufficient preliminary evidence to justify the very large randomised controlled trials required to establish whether the use of these tests will reduce mortality. Three such trials are currently recruiting volunteers: in the UK, Europe and the USA.

1

Test requirements in ovarian cancer screening

As well as being acceptable and affordable, a screening test must have high sensitivity (the probability of the test being positive in individuals with the disease) and high specificity (the probability of the test being negative in patients without the disease). High sensitivity is crucial in order to maximise the potential for influencing survival. High specificity is necessary, as the end result of a false positive result is likely to be surgery. It is unlikely that either clinicians or the public would be willing to accept a test which results in many women undergoing unnecessary laparotomies for each case of ovarian cancer detected. Because the disease is relatively uncommon, a screening test for the post-menopausal population would require 99.6 per cent specificity in order to detect one case of ovarian cancer for every 10 women testing positive (i.e. a positive predictive value of 10 per cent) (Jacobs & Oram 1988). Lower specificity will achieve a positive predictive value of 10 per cent in high-risk populations. For example, a specificity of only 92 per cent would be acceptable for screening BRCA1 gene carriers, as the incidence of ovarian cancer in this group is far greater than in the general population (Jacobs & Oram 1988).

Tests for the early detection of ovarian cancer

Non-ultrasound-based imaging

High-technology imaging modalities (CT, MRI, radioimmunoscintigraphy) are not practical for mass screening but may be able to define the malignant status of an ovary which produces abnormal levels of tumour markers or appears abnormal on ultrasound scanning, thus improving the overall positive predictive value of a screening strategy. Radioimmunoscintigraphy utilises the preferential binding of specific antibodies to a target tissue. The SM3 monoclonal antibody (Jobling *et al.* 1990), which binds to malignant ovarian tissue 17 times more efficiently than benign tissue, is currently being evaluated as part of the large randomised controlled trial of ovarian cancer screening at St Bartholomew's Hospital.

Complementary tumour markers

CA 125 is the only tumour marker to have been used prospectively in large studies of ovarian cancer screening, but combinations of tumour markers able to complement each other have the potential to improve sensitivity and specificity. Promising candidate markers which complement CA 125 include OVX-1 and M-CSF (Woolas *et al.* 1993), CA-72-4 (Jacobs *et al.* 1993b) and CYFRA-21 (Inaba *et al.* 1995). Preliminary data from our own laboratory suggest that OVX-1 may be unstable unless serum is separated soon after venepuncture and this has important implications if samples for population screening are to be sent by post to a central laboratory. Emerging neural network technology may further enhance the sensitivity and specificity of multiple markers by enabling sophisticated interpretation of marker levels relative to each other.

Ultrasound

Transabdominal ultrasound was investigated prospectively in 5,540 women by Campbell *et al.* (1989). Although five ovarian cancers were detected, all of which were stage Ia, three of them were borderline (and therefore unlikely to have caused death if left undetected). In addition, the specificity of this study was only 94.6 per cent and consequently approximately 50 women underwent surgery for each case of ovarian cancer detected. The University of Kentucky study (van Nagell *et al.* 1995) investigated transvaginal ultrasound in 8,500 asymptomatic women: of these, 121 underwent surgery, of whom eight had invasive ovarian cancer (6 stage Ia, 1 stage IIc and 1 stage IIIb). The sensitivity was 88.8 per cent and 15 women were operated on for every case of ovarian cancer detected. The specificity of transvaginal ultrasound may be improved by use of a morphological index which scores the scans by parameters such as tumour volume, wall structure and septal structure. However, women with masses which appear benign according to a morphological index need careful follow-up to assess any change in the mass, and this makes surgery hard to avoid. Colour flow Doppler to assess the presence and distribution of low-resistance neovasculature in malignant ovaries may also increase specificity. Kurjak *et al.* (1992) scanned 1,000 women transvaginally and performed Doppler on women with abnormal scans. They detected 27 out of 29 ovarian cancers, and sensitivity and specificity were 96 per cent and 95 per cent respectively. However, 257 women in this study were symptomatic, and 25 of the 29 malignancies occurred in this group, so these results cannot be extrapolated to predict the performance of Doppler in a mass-screening programme. Bourne *et al.* (1991) screened 1,601 self-referred women with a family history of ovarian cancer. They detected three borderline and three invasive (2 stage Ia and 1 stage III) cancers, and approximately ten women were operated on for each case of ovarian cancer detected. Retrospectively applying Doppler and morphological index criteria resulted in an increase in specificity such that only two women would have had surgery for each case of ovarian cancer detected. However, sensitivity would have been reduced to only 60 per cent. More recently, Kurjak *et al.* (1994) reported the results of transvaginal Doppler screening of 5,013 women. Of these, 38 were operated on for four cases of ovarian cancer (2 stage Ia and 2 stage Ib), giving a positive predictive value of 10.5 per cent. However, true and false negative rates were not reported in this study, so it is impossible to comment on sensitivity and specificity. Ultrasound screening has not yet achieved the level of specificity required for screening the general population. It is also fairly expensive and intrusive, compared with venepuncture for tumour markers. In addition, it relies upon highly skilled operators, making quality control a potential problem.

CA 125

The tumour-associated antigen CA 125 was first detected using a murine monoclonal antibody, generated in response to immunological challenge with an ovarian cancer cell line. Discovered by Bast *et al.* (1981), it has been found to be elevated in the serum of 80–85 per cent of women with epithelial ovarian cancer (Jacobs & Bast 1989). Apparently, healthy post-menopausal women with a level of ≥30 U/ml have a 35.9-fold increased risk of a clinical diagnosis of ovarian cancer within one year (Jacobs *et al.* 1996). CA 125 is not usually elevated in the early stages of non-epithelial ovarian malignancies, but is elevated in a variety of other conditions, including endometriosis (Pittaway & Fayez 1986) and various symptomatic malignancies (Haga *et al.* 1986). In general, any condition which causes inflammation of a mesothelial surface (i.e. peritoneum, pleura or pericardium) can cause a rise in serum CA 125. This lack of specificity for ovarian cancer is potentially problematic, as a false positive screen may result in unnecessary surgery. However, most causes of an elevated CA 125 are either rare in post-menopausal women (who would be the target for population screening) or are clinically apparent. Furthermore, retrospective use of a mathematical algorithm (Skates *et al.* 1995) which analysed rates of change of CA 125, during a sequential screening study involving 5,500 women, had a sensitivity of 83 per cent and a specificity of 99.7 per cent for detecting ovarian cancer in the year following the last screen. These encouraging results reflect the finding that women with ovarian cancer tend to have CA 125 levels which continually rise, while those with other conditions tend to have static or fluctuating levels. Our own unit has demonstrated that use of this algorithm improves the operating characteristics of CA 125 so that both sensitivity and specificity can be maximised. We are therefore using the algorithm as the primary test in the St Bartholomew's randomised controlled trial of ovarian cancer screening.

Multimodal screening

The largest reported screening trial (Jacobs *et al.* 1993a) involved 22,000 post-menopausal women over 45 years old. The population was screened with CA 125 and then proceeded to ultrasound only if their CA 125 was ≥30 U/ml. This multimodal approach had a specificity of 99.9 per cent, a positive predictive value of 26.8 per cent and an apparent sensitivity of 78.6 per cent after one year of follow-up. We are combining this multimodal approach with the mathematical algorithm described above in the St Bartholomew's Hospital randomised controlled trial: 120,000 women will be recruited over three years and randomised to screening or follow-up for a mean of six years. The screened group will have annual CA 125 testing and those with intermediate results will have a repeat test at 1–6 months, while those with a high-risk result will have a transvaginal ultrasound scan. Women with scans suggestive of malignancy or rapidly rising CA 125 levels will be investigated surgically. This study has 80 per cent power to detect a 30 per cent reduction in mortality from ovarian cancer in the screened group. A pilot study of 10,000 women screened for a year resulted in 15 women undergoing surgery, of whom three had ovarian cancer (one stage Ic, one stage IIa and one stage Ia borderline).

Which population should be screened?

The general population

Although results from studies involving ultrasound and/or CA 125 have proved encouraging and indicate that pre-clinical ovarian cancer can be detected, no definitive randomised trial of screening for ovarian cancer has yet been completed. Until data from the three major trials currently recruiting have matured, it is impossible to know whether screening will save lives. The incidence of ovarian cancer necessitates very large numbers of subjects and long-term follow-up in these studies. Consequently, results of the first trial to be completed are not expected before 2005. Until that time, the value of general population screening will remain uncertain. Screening this group cannot currently be recommended as it exposes women to potential anxiety and the risk of unnecessary surgery, with no guarantee of a survival benefit if they do develop ovarian cancer.

The high-risk population

The situation for women at very high risk of ovarian cancer may be different. The specificity requirements in such women are less stringent than those for the general population, because of their higher incidence of ovarian cancer. Both ultrasound and CA 125 have already demonstrated adequate specificity to achieve an acceptable positive predictive value for the detection of pre-clinical disease in this group (Jacobs & Oram 1988). Although no screening method has so far been shown to reduce mortality, screening is frequently offered to young women with a strong family history of breast and ovarian cancer. Women in this situation should be counselled about the risks and unproven benefits of screening, so that they can make informed decisions about their management. The UK Central Coordinating Committee for Cancer Research is currently recruiting 3,000 women at high risk to a prospective study involving screening with both CA 125 and ultrasound. It is hoped that analysis of these data will lead to the development of an optimal screening strategy for women at high risk of ovarian cancer.

5

The acceptability of screening

As with other forms of cancer screening, socio-economic and demographic factors may influence screening uptake; the University of Kentucky screening programme found that educated women living close to the screening location were the most likely to attend (Pavlik *et al.* 1995). Women with a family history of the disease are also more likely to attend if they are in employment and admit to being concerned about their risk (Schwartz *et al.* 1995). Lower screening uptake among lower-income women has provided cause for concern. However, unlike the situation in cervical cancer, the prevalence of ovarian cancer is not associated with lower socio-economic class (Beral *et al.* 1978). Age and race were found to play a role in an English study (Wolfe & Raju 1994) which found that women aged over 65 and Caucasians were less willing to be screened. These data suggest that screening may be more acceptable to higher-risk populations and that mass ovarian screening may suffer from uptake problems similar to those of breast and cervical screening programmes. Nevertheless, it is encouraging that 98.7 per cent of 22,000 women complied with follow-up at one year in a sequential multimodal screening study (Pavlik *et al.* 1995).

The psychological impact of screening

There are no published data on the psychological impact of screening the general population for ovarian cancer, although some work on screening high-risk groups has been reported. Psychological distress and worries about cancer fell significantly following a scan showing no abnormalities in an UK-based familial ovarian cancer screening programme (Wardle *et al.* 1993). Following a positive scan, distress increased most in those with an information-seeking coping style and those who were referred for surgery. Anxiety levels returned to baseline in all patients following surgery. However, all surgery yielded benign diagnoses and this study spanned only one round of testing. Evidence is accumulating that variations in coping strategies may determine an individual's emotional response to screening (Basen-Engquist 1997), and anxiety and depression scores of those who consider themselves at high risk by virtue of a family history may be particularly high (Erlick Robinson *et al.* 1997). The randomised controlled trials of ovarian cancer screening will provide an important opportunity to study the psychological impact of screening on the general population. Such studies may have major implications for mass screening.

Cost–benefit analysis of ovarian cancer screening

If ovarian cancer screening is shown to save lives, then before it can be implemented on a large scale, governments and/or health insurers will demand evidence of cost-effectiveness. Reliable data on this aspect of screening will become available as a result of the ongoing randomised controlled trials of screening in the general population. Currently, the literature on this subject is sparse, and what work there is consists of estimates from computer modelling. This research must be interpreted with caution, particularly with regards to the absolute costs. However, one can at least use such work for comparing the costs of different screening strategies. A meta-analysis (Holbert 1994) has suggested that using CA 125 and ultrasound concurrently would cost $445,177 per case of stage I ovarian cancer found. This would translate as a total cost of $14 billion to screen all women aged over 45 years in the USA, suggesting that ultrasound will be too costly to use as a primary screening test for the general population. Urban *et al.* (1997) modelled the probable cost per year of life saved of various screening strategies. In this model, a sequential multimodal strategy was the most cost-effective method of mass screening over a wide range of assumptions about test costs and performance. A cost of $51,000 per year of life saved was achieved using annual CA 125 screening as a primary test, prompting a transvaginal ultrasound scan only if the level either doubled since the previous screen or was ≥35 U/ml. This cost is comparable to the estimates of cost per year of life saved for breast cancer screening (Mandelblatt 1997). At present, the most cost-effective approach to ovarian cancer screening would appear to be a multimodal strategy, using CA 125 as a primary test and ultrasound as a secondary test in those women who have an abnormal CA 125 result. Such a strategy is also likely to have an acceptable positive predictive value (Jacobs 1993a).

Conclusions

Ovarian cancer screening outside of the context of a randomised controlled trial cannot currently be recommended for the general population, because of unproven efficacy. However, women at high risk of ovarian cancer, by virtue of a proven germ-line mutation in a predisposing gene or a strong family history of ovarian and/or breast cancer, may benefit from current screening technologies. Anyone undergoing screening should be made aware that it has not yet been proven to reduce mortality. Screening also exposes women to the possibility of anxiety and unnecessary surgery, with its attendant morbidity and (rarely) mortality. In the future, screening test performance may be improved by the use of novel complementary markers and further optimised using neural networks. Genetic screening may facilitate more accurate definition of high-risk populations and imaging technologies such as radioimmunoscintigraphy may improve overall positive predictive value, thus limiting the numbers of women requiring surgical investigation. Ongoing randomised trials of screening in the general population and studies analysing data on screening and outcome in high-risk women should provide important information during the next decade.

References

Basen-Engquist K (1997). Ovarian cancer screening and psychosocial issues: relevance to clinical practice. *Gynecol Oncol* **65**, 195–6.

Bast R, Klug T L, St John E *et al.* (1981). Reactivity of a monoclonal antibody with human ovarian carcinoma. *J Clin Invest* **68**, 1331–7.

Beral V, Fraser P & Chilvers C (1978). Does pregnancy protect against ovarian cancer? *Lancet* **1**, 1083–7.

Bourne T H, Whitehead M I, Campbell S *et al.* (1991). Ultrasound screening for familial ovarian cancer. *Gynecol Oncol* **43**, 92–7.

Campbell S, Bhan V, Royston P *et al.* (1989). Transabdominal ultrasound screening for ovarian cancer. *Brit Med J* **299**, 1363–7.

Erlick Robinson G, Rosen B P, Bradley L N, Rockert WG, Carr M L, Cole D E & Murphy K J (1997). Psychological impact of screening for familial ovarian cancer: reactions to initial assessment. *Gynecol Oncol* **65**,197–205.

Haga Y, Sakamoto K, Egami H *et al.* (1986). Clinical significance of serum CA 125 values in patients with cancers of the digestive system. *Am J Med Sci* **292**, 30–4.

Holbert TR (1994). Screening transvaginal ultrasonography of postmenopausal women in a private office setting. *Am J Obstet Gynecol* **170**, 1699–704.

Inaba N, Negishi Y, Fukasawa I *et al.* (1995). Cytokeratin fragment 21-1 in gynecologic malignancy: comparison with cancer antigen 125 and squamous cell carcinoma-related antigen. *Tumour Biol* **16**(6), 345–52.

Jacobs I & Oram D (1988). Screening for ovarian cancer. *Biomed and Pharmacother* **42**, 589–96.

Jacobs I J & Bast R C (1989). The CA 125 tumour-associated antigen: a review of the literature. *Hum Reprod* **4**, 1–12.

Jacobs I, Davies A P, Bridges J *et al.* (1993a). Prevalence screening for ovarian cancer in post-menopausal women by CA 125 measurement and ultrasonography. *Brit Med J* **306**, 1030–4.

Jacobs I J, Rivera H, Oram D H & Bast R C Jr (1993b). Differential diagnosis of ovarian cancer with tumour markers CA 125, CA 15-3 and TAG 72.3. *Br J Obstet Gynecol* **100**(12), 1120–4.

Jacobs I J, Skates S, Prys Davis A *et al.* (1996). Risk of diagnosis of ovarian cancer after raised serum CA 125 concentration: a prospective cohort study. *Brit Med J* **313**, 1355–8.

Jobling T W, Granowska M & Britton K E (1990). Radioimmunoscintigraphy of ovarian tumours using a new monoclonal antibody, SM3. *Gynecol Oncol* **38**, 468–72.

Kurjak A, Schulman H, Sosic A *et al.* (1992). Transvaginal ultrasound, color flow, and Doppler waveform of the postmenopausal adnexal mass. *Obstet Gynecol* **80**, 917–21.

Kurjak A, Shalan H, Kupesic S *et al.* (1994). An attempt to screen asymptomatic women for ovarian cancer with transvaginal color and pulsed Doppler sonography. *J Ultrasound Med* **13**, 295–301.

Mandelblatt J, Freeman H, Winczewski D *et al.* (1997). The cost and effects of cervical and breast cancer screening in a public hospital emergency room. *Amer J Public Health* **8**, 1182–9.

Nguyen N H, Averette H E, Hoskins W *et al.* (1993). National survey of ovarian carcinoma VI. Critical assessment of current International Federation of Obstetrics and Gynaecology staging system. *Cancer* **72**, 3007–11.

OPCS (1994). *Cancer statistics registrations 1989.* MB1. HMSO, London.

Pavlik E J, van Nagell J R, DePriest P D *et al.* (1995). Participation in transvaginal ovarian cancer screening: compliance, correlation factors, and costs. *Gynecol Oncol* **57**, 395–400.

Pittaway D E & Fayez J A (1986). The use of CA-125 in the diagnosis and management of endometriosis. *Fertil Steril* **46**, 790–5.

Schwartz M, Lerman C, Daly M *et al.* (1995). Utilization of ovarian cancer screening by women at increased risk. *Cancer Epidemiol Biomarkers Prev* **4**, 269–73.

Skates S J, Xu F J, Yu Y H *et al.* (1995). Toward an optimal algorithm for ovarian cancer screening with longitudinal tumor markers. *Cancer* **76**, 2004–10.

Urban N, Drescher C, Etzioni R & Colby C (1997). Use of a stochastic simulation model to identify an efficient protocol for ovarian cancer screening. *Controlled Clinical Trials* **18**, 251–70.

van der Burg M E L, van Lent M, Buyse M *et al.* (1995). The effect of debulking surgery after induction chemotherapy on the prognosis in advanced epithelial ovarian cancer. *NEJM* **332**, 629–34.

van Nagell J R, Gallion H D, Pavlik E J *et al.* (1995). Ovarian cancer screening. *Cancer* **76**, 2086–91.

Wardle F J, Collins W, Pernet A L *et al.* (1993). Psychological impact of screening for familial ovarian cancer. *J Natl Cancer Inst* **85**, 653–7.

Wolfe C D & Raju K S (1994). The attitudes of women and feasibility of screening for ovarian and endometrial cancers in inner city practices. *Eur J Obstet Gynecol Reprod Biol* **56**, 117–20.

Woolas R P, Xu F J, Jacobs I J *et al.* (1993). Elevation of multiple serum markers in patients with stage I ovarian cancer. *J Natl Cancer Inst* **85**, 1748–51.

Errata

p. 2, line 4 from bottom, *for* CA-72-4 *read* CA 15-3
p. 6, line 17 from top, *for* (Pavlik *et al.* 1995) *read* (Jacobs *et al.* 1993a)

Chapter 2

Current management of ovarian cancer in the UK – problems and potential

S B Kaye

Introduction

Over the past 20 years there has been a definite, albeit modest, improvement in the overall outcome of treatment for ovarian cancer. As a study by Berrino *et al.* (1995) shows, the gap between incidence and mortality in Europe, particularly in younger women, is gradually becoming wider. Two questions arise: (a) why is this, and (b) how can we do better?

The answer to question (a) is uncertain, but the reason is likely to be a combination of two factors. First, the use of platinum-based therapy, particularly carboplatin, has been shown in a large-scale study in Scotland (Junor *et al.* 1994) to be an independent factor determining outcome, and its introduction on a wide scale is likely to be an important factor. Second, there is more recognition of the importance of optimal initial surgery – the problem is now partly one of its widespread implementation. So, what is the answer to question (b)?

How can we do better?

The overall aim is to maximise the number of patients achieving a complete remission after initial therapy, and to identify the best method for preventing relapse. The following sections consider the posed question under three headings:

- surgery
- chemotherapy
- novel treatments resulting from laboratory research.

Surgery

Issues which are most important include:

- *Who should do it?* Data from the Scottish audit (Junor *et al.* 1994) indicate a better outcome if initial surgery is carried out by a gynaecologist rather than a general surgeon, independent of other factors. More recently, data suggest that survival is better for patients operated on by a specialist gynaecologist rather than a generalist (E. Junor, personal communication), and clearly there are important implications for the organisation of clinical services. Data such as these have led directly to the generation of clinical guidelines, the implementation of which is attracting increasing attention.

- *What operations/what is its optimal timing?* Initial cytoreduction remains the most widely accepted goal of the definitive first operation, although exactly how far that procedure should go in attempting to remove all disease is a matter of conjecture. Many patients do not have the benefit of this initial major tumour bulk reduction, but a randomised trial (van der Burg *et al.* 1995) has shown a significant survival benefit for interval debulking, i.e. repeat surgery after three courses of chemotherapy. This trial has had considerable impact, with many centres, particularly in Europe, opting for this procedure as a preferred option in patients who did not have optimal debulking initially. Others point out that the results of one trial need to be confirmed before it can be widely adopted as standard practice, and in fact a confirmatory trial in the UK is now under way under the aegis of the MRC.

- *What is its role in the relapse setting?* Here there is a major dearth of information from randomised trials. Retrospective data (Berek 1999) would suggest that surgery to resect isolated recurrences may be beneficial for patients in good general condition with a relatively long interval since prior chemotherapy. However, this needs to be confirmed in a randomised trial, such as the one planned by the European Organisation for Research and Treatment of Cancer (EORTC). An important endpoint, as well as survival, is quality of life; does surgery for relapse lead to a measurable improvement in a situation in which palliation of symptoms is ultimately the primary aim?

Chemotherapy

Results from two major trials in advanced ovarian cancer, i.e. GOG 111 in the USA (McGuire *et al.* 1996), and OV-10, the Intergroup study (Stuart *et al.* 1998), indicate that the two-drug combination of paclitaxel-cisplatin is significantly superior to the previous standard regime of cyclophosphamide and cisplatin. The benefit is seen in progression-free and, interestingly, even more in overall survival, with a 12-month overall survival difference which was virtually identical in the two trials. This improvement over previous treatment is of a similar scale to that which it has been calculated could be attributed to the introduction of cisplatin itself over 20 years ago (Dembo 1986). Thus, paclitaxel is now recommended for first-line combination therapy; within the UK this has led to considerable problems relating to its cost, and these are only gradually being resolved.

The introduction of paclitaxel-cisplatin has raised many questions. These include:

• *Is the other taxoid, docetaxel, an alternative candidate for first-line combination chemotherapy?* Phase II trials have indicated (Kaye *et al.* 1997) that, as a single agent, docetaxel has activity in refractory patients at least equivalent to that of paclitaxel, with a response rate of 28 per cent. A feasibility study of docetaxel-carboplatin in first-line treatment (Vasey *et al.* 1998) has indicated that this is a well-tolerated and active regime, with a 'platelet-sparing' effect similar to that seen with paclitaxel, but with a very low level of neurotoxicity.

• *Can carboplatin now replace cisplatin in first-line chemotherapy?* The results of a number of randomised trials, recently updated in a large-scale meta-analysis (Advanced Ovarian Cancer Trialists Group 1998), show no difference in outcome between regimes containing carboplatin and cisplatin. These trials pre-dated paclitaxel combinations, but the two randomised trials of paclitaxel-carboplatin versus paclitaxel-cisplatin analysed so far (du Bois *et al.* 1998; Neijt *et al.* 1998) also show no significant difference. Although a minority of investigators still prefer to wait for mature survival data, the superior toxicity profile of carboplatin has convinced many clinicians to switch from cisplatin at this stage.

• *What is the optimal duration of therapy?* Although previous randomised trials appear to indicate no benefit for continuing chemotherapy beyond six cycles, these trials are, to an extent, flawed because of a high drop-out rate. In any case more extended chemotherapy may be more relevant to taxoid-containing regimes, and randomised trials involving these new regimes are certainly warranted.

• *Should the taxoid and platinum drugs be given together or sequentially?* All the completed and current randomised trials of first-line therapy involving taxoid/platinum regimes have used combinations in which both components are given together. It is conceivable that sequential therapy may be efficacious since different populations of cells may be targeted. For instance, ovarian cancer cells with mutations of p53 which are generally resistant to platinum may be sensitive, even hypersensitive, to taxoids (Neijt *et al.* 1998). Sequential regimes, involving either single agents or new combinations, clearly merit further study.

• *Is the addition of other new drugs worthwhile?* Ovarian cancer has been a productive area for the identification of new cytotoxic agents, and these are listed in Table 2.1. In each case, 'activity' has been seen in patients with refractory disease, including those who have progressed on prior therapy with paclitaxel. This activity is generally in the 15–30 per cent response rate range, and the challenge in future years will be to incorporate the most promising of these agents with first-line therapy. As before, this may well involve the development of new sequential regimens, perhaps taking advantage of information gained at interventional surgery.

Table 2.1 New cytotoxic agents

Agent	No. of patients	Response rate (%)	Reference
Topotecan	96	23	Huinink *et al.* (1997)
Gemcitabine	51	16	Lund *et al.* (1994)
Oral VP16	41	27	Rose *et al.* (1998)
Liposomal doxorubicin	35	20	Muggia *et al.* (1997)
Navelbine	38	29	Burger *et al.* (1996)
Oxaliplatin	18	29	Chollet *et al.* (1994)

• *Who pays?* A key issue in the introduction of a new cytotoxic agent, particularly in the UK, is cost. New drug development is an expensive undertaking, and so new agents will generally be considerably more costly than those in current usage: this is certainly the case for paclitaxel. However, overall expenditure on cytotoxic drugs in the UK is extremely modest; in fact, it is one of the lowest in Europe. Purchasers of health care will always need to make choices when new treatments are developed, but usually evidence of clear survival benefit in cancer treatment is sufficient to convince them.

Novel treatments resulting from laboratory research

Most clinicians agree that the major hurdle to overcome in ovarian cancer is the development of drug resistance. The challenge is to understand the mechanisms which underlie this process in the clinic. Numerous laboratory studies have identified a range of possibilities, in experimental ovarian cancer models of both platinum and taxoid resistance. A few are listed in Table 2.2, and several others are also candidates. The main issue is one of clinical relevance, and here the need for more translational studies is a high priority. A limited amount of data point to mutations of p53 as a clinically important event (Righetti *et al.* 1996); studies in our own laboratory are currently focusing on mismatch repair deficiency, specifically loss of hMLH1 expression, as a mechanism which could explain resistance to a range of agents (Strathdee *et al.* 1999).

Table 2.2 Mechanisms underlying drug resistance in ovarian cancer

Drug	Mechanism	Reference
Platinum	p53 mutations	Brown (1996)
Platinum and alkylating agents	Enhanced DNA repair	van der Zee & DeVries (1996)
Multiple	Mismatch repair deficiency	Fink *et al.* (1998)
Taxoids	P-glycoprotein (multidrug resistance)	van der Zee *et al.* (1995)
Taxoids	Increased bcl-2 (and Raf-1-kinase) activity	Rasouli Nia *et al.* (1998)

The development of new therapeutic strategies aimed at circumventing drug resistance is an area of very active research. These include agents targeting the p53 mutant cell (e.g. the Onyx 015 virus (Heise *et al.* 1991)), genetic therapy aimed at replacing wild-type p53 function (Roth *et al.* 1996), P-glycoprotein-modulators (e.g. PSC833 (Boesch *et al.* 1991)), and a range of modulators of cell signalling. Mismatch repair deficiency may well be approached using hypomethylating agents, or by identifying agents which are active in mismatch repair deficiency models (e.g. oxaliplatin (Raymond *et al.* 1998)).

Other new targets include tumour angiogenesis, and it seems likely that most of the agents developed with these targets in mind will find their optimal role in combination with or following conventional chemotherapy.

Conclusions

In summary, advances are being made in ovarian cancer management, but these are slow, and further improvements are clearly essential and are expected.

The challenges now are: (a) to ensure that all ovarian cancer patients have access to best quality multidisciplinary care, and (b) to ensure proper dialogue between clinicians and laboratory scientists, so that advances in understanding can lead to improvements in treatment without delay.

References

Advanced Ovarian Cancer Trialists Group (1998). Chemotherapy in advanced ovarian cancer: four systematic meta-analyses from 37 individual trials. *Br J Cancer* **78**, 1479–87.

Berek J S (1998). Surgery during chemotherapy and at relapse of ovarian cancer. *Ann Oncol* **10**, (Suppl.1), 3–8.

Berrino F, Sant M, Verdecchia A, Capocaccia R, Hakulinen T & Estéfe J (1995). *Survival of cancer patients in Europe: a EUROCARE study.* IARC Scientific Publications, Lyon (pp.292–304).

Boesch D, Gaveriaux C, Jachez B, Pourtiermanzanedo A, Bollinger P & Loor F (1991). *In vivo* circumvention of P-glycoprotein-mediated multidrug resistance of tumor-cells with SDZ PSC-833. *Cancer Res* **51**, 4226–33.

Brown R (1996). Cellular responses to DNA damage and cisplatin resistance. In *Ovarian cancer 4* (ed. F Sharp, T Blackett, R Leake & J Berek), pp.205–13. Chapman and Hall, London.

Burger R A, Bowman S, White R *et al.* (1996). Phase II trial of navelbine in advanced epithelial ovarian cancer. *Proc Amer Soc Clin Oncol* **15**, 286.

Chollet P, Bensmaine M, Deloche C *et al.* (1994). Preliminary results of phase II study of oxaliplatin: a new active agent in platinum pretreated ovarian cancer. *Ann Oncol* **5** (Suppl.8), 110.

Dembo A J (1986). Controversy over combination chemotherapy in advanced ovarian cancer: what we learn from reports of matured data. *J Clin Oncol* **4**, 1573–6.

du Bois A, Richter B, Warm M *et al.* (1998). Cisplatin/paclitaxel vs carboplatin/paclitaxel as 1st-line treatment in ovarian cancer. *Proc Amer Soc Clin Oncol* **17**, 1395.

Fink D, Aebi S & Howell S (1998). The role of DNA mismatch repair in drug resistance. *Clin Cancer Res* **4**, 1–6.

Heise C, Sampson Johannes A, Williams A, McCormick F, VonHoff D D & Kirn D H (1997). ONYX-015, an E1B gene-attenuated adenovirus, causes tumor-specific cytolysis and antitumoral efficacy that can be augmented by standard chemotherapeutic agents. *Nature Med* **3**, 639–45.

Huinink W T B, Gore M, Carmichael J *et al.* (1997). Topotecan versus paclitaxel for the treatment of recurrent epithelial ovarian cancer. *J Clin Oncol* **15**, 2183–93.

Junor E J, Hole D J & Gillis CR (1994). Management of ovarian cancer – referral to a multidisciplinary team matters. *Br J Cancer* **70**, 363–70.

Kaye S B, Piccart M, Aapro M, Francis P & Kavanagh J (1997). Phase II trials of docetaxel (Taxotere®) in advanced ovarian cancer – an updated overview. *Eur J Cancer* **33**, 2167–70.

Lund B, Hansen O P, Theilade K *et al.* (1994). Phase II study of gemcitabine in previously treated ovarian cancer patients. *J Natl Cancer Ins* **86**, 1530–3.

McGuire W P, Hoskins W J, Brady M F *et al.* (1996). Cyclophosphamide and cisplatin compared with paclitaxel and cisplatin in patients with stage III and stage IV ovarian cancer. *N Engl J Med* **334**, 1–6.

Muggia F M, Hainsworth J D & Jeffers S (1997). Phase II study of liposomal doxorubicin in refractory ovarian cancer: antitumour activity and toxicity modification by liposomal encapsulation. *J Clin Oncol* **15**, 987–93.

Neijt J P, Engelholm S A, Tuxen M *et al.* (1998). Paclitaxel-cisplatin vs paclitaxel-carboplatin in previously untreated ovarian cancer. *Ann Oncol* **9** (Suppl.4), 65.

15

Rasouli Nia A, Liu D, Perdue S & Britten R A (1998). High Raf-1 kinase activity protects human tumor cells against paclitaxel-induced cytotoxicity. *Clin Cancer Res* **4**, 1111–16.

Righetti S C, Della Torre G, Pilotti, S *et al.* (1996). A comparative study of p53 gene mutations, protein accumulation, and response to cisplatin-based chemotherapy in advanced ovarian carcinoma. *Cancer Res* **56**, 689–93.

Rose P G, Blessing J A, Mayer A & Homesley H D (1998). Prolonged oral etoposide as second-line therapy for platinum-resistant and platinum-sensitive ovarian carcinoma: a Gynecologic Oncology Group Study. *J Clin Oncol* **16**, 405–10.

Roth J A, Nguyen D, Lawrence D D *et al.* (1996). Retrovirus-mediated wild-type p53 gene-transfer to tumors of patients with lung-cancer. *Nature Med* **2**, 985–91.

Strathdee G, MacKean M, Illand M & Brown R (1999). A role for methylation of the hMLH1 promoter in loss of hMLH1 expression and drug resistance in ovarian cancer. *Oncogene* **18**, 2335–41.

Stuart G, Bertelsen K, Mangioni C *et al.* (1998). Updated analysis shows a highly significant improved survival, with cisplatin-paclitaxel as first-line treatment of advanced ovarian cancer: mature results of the Intergroup trial. *Proc Amer Soc Clin Oncol* **17**, 1394.

van der Burg M, van Lent M, Buyse M *et al.* (1995). The effect of debulking surgery after induction chemotherapy on the prognosis in advanced ovarian cancer. *New Engl J Med* **332**, 629–34.

van der Zee A, & DeVries EG (1996). Drug resistance factors. In *Ovarian cancer 4* (ed. F Sharp, T Blackett, R Leake & J Berek), pp.221–33. Chapman & Hall, London.

van der Zee AG, Hollema H, Swurmeier AJ *et al.* (1995). The value of P-glycoprotein, glutathione-S-transferase, C-erbB-2 and p53 as prognostic factors in ovarian carcinomas. *J Clin Oncol* **13**, 70–8.

Vasey PA, Atkinson R, Coleman R *et al.* (1998). Preliminary report of a dose-finding study of a docetaxel-carboplatin combination in untreated advanced epithelial ovarian cancer (EOC). *Proc Amer Soc Clin Oncol* **17**, 349a.

Wahl A, Donaldson K, Fairchild C *et al.* (1996). Loss of normal p53 function confers sensitization to Taxol. *Nature Med* **2**, 72–8.

Chapter 3

Who should treat ovarian cancer? Challenging the perceived wisdom

Sean Kehoe

Introduction

Ovarian cancer affects approximately 5,000 women each year in England and Wales, with an annual death rate of 4,500, making it the fourth most common cause of death from malignancy in women (OPCS 1993). Policy changes in cancer services and, in particular, the proposals of the Calman/Hine report (Department of Health 1995) have addressed the principal issues relating to the ideal configuration of cancer services required to optimise survival patterns. While the primary contact for a woman with suspected ovarian cancer is most often a general gynaecologist, there are now specialist gynaecological oncologists available. Within the fields of medical and clinical oncology, there are specialists who have a particular interest in managing ovarian cancer. However, these are but two groups of specialists involved in treating ovarian cancer and many others, such as the family doctor, palliative care specialists, pathologists, dieticians, Macmillan nurses and psychologists have equally important contributions to make to patient care, and together form the multidisciplinary team. This chapter attempts to answer the posed question – namely, 'Who should treat ovarian cancer?' – with available evidence from the literature.

The surgeon

The diagnosis and staging of ovarian carcinoma requires a laparotomy. The elements relating to appropriate staging are shown in Box 3.1 and it is reasonable to expect that those operating on patients with ovarian carcinoma have the required surgical skills to undertake the necessary procedures. The recommended surgical intervention is a total abdominal hysterectomy, bilateral salpingo-oophorectomy, omentectomy and 'debulking' of tumour (Department of Health 1991). Total macroscopic excision of all intra-abdominal disease should be the main objective of surgery, but in many cases this is not feasible and tumour debulking is advised (Boente *et al.* 1998). Although debate on the true impact of 'debulking' disease in ovarian cancer will persist until completion of an appropriate clinical trial, this approach remains part of standard therapy (Kehoe 1996). To achieve optimum debulking, bowel resection and other surgical procedures not normally considered within the brief of general gynaecological training may be required. Hence, the evolution of gynaecological oncology specialists.

Box 3.1 FIGO staging for ovarian carcinoma

Stage I
Growth limited to the ovaries

- *Stage Ia:* Growth limited to one ovary, no ascites, no tumour on external surface, capsule intact
- *Stage Ib:* Growth limited to both ovaries, no ascites, no tumour on external surface, capsule intact
- *Stage Ic:* Stage Ia or Ib but with tumour on the surface of one or both ovaries, or with capsule rupture, or with ascites present containing malignant cells or with positive peritoneal washings

Stage II
Growth involving one or both
ovaries with pelvic extension

- *Stage IIa:* Extension and/or metastases to the uterus and/or tubes
- *Stage IIb:* Extension to other pelvic tissues
- *Stage IIc:* Stage IIa or IIb but with tumour on the surface of one or both ovaries, or with capsule(s) rupture, or with ascites present containing malignant cells or with positive peritoneal washings

Stage III
Extra-pelvic tumour present

- *Stage IIIa:* Tumour grossly limited to the true pelvis with negative retroperitoneal/inguinal nodes but with histologically confirmed microscopic seeding of abdominal peritoneal surfaces
- *Stage IIIb:* Tumour involving one or both ovaries with histologically confirmed implants of abdominal peritoneal surfaces none exceeding 2 cm in diameter. Nodes are negative
- *Stage IIIc:* Abdominal implants greater than 2 cm in diameter and/or positive retroperitoneal or inguinal nodes

Stage IV
Growth involving one or both
ovaries with distant metastases

If pleural effusion is present, there must be positive cytology to allocate stage IV. Parenchymal liver metastases equals stage IV.

[*Source:* Pettersson (1988)]

Arguably, one could suggest that a gynaecologist in conjunction with a general surgeon would achieve a similar goal as the gynaecological oncologist. However, within the literature, such co-operation does not seem evident. Indeed, a large epidemiological study in the West Midlands revealed that a third of women had primary operations by a general surgeon with a significantly poorer survival, compared with those operated on by a gynaecologist (Kehoe *et al.* 1994). This has been supported by a subsequent study by Woodman *et al.* (1997), and while accepting that many unaccounted variables may have contributed to these findings, the fact remains that outcome will probably be improved by virtue of a gynaecologist's involvement. Evidence indicating that gynaecologists rather than general surgeons should undertake care seems reasonably demonstrated.

Regarding the potential advantage of a gynaecological oncologist over a general gynaecologist, the evidence is circumstantial. However, that which is, favours the oncology-trained specialist. For example, gynaecological oncologists achieve a greater proportion of patients optimally debulked (Eisenkop *et al.* 1992; Nguyen *et al.* 1993), although this is not reflected in survival patterns, as shown by a multicentre US study (Roohan *et al.* 1998). Information from other cancers, such as breast and colorectal, has indicated the superior outcome with patients cared for by surgeons with a high volume of cases (Selby *et al.* 1996). Intuition would suggest that those surgeons familiar with managing ovarian cancer are the most likely group to achieve optimum survival – a somewhat logical conclusion. However, to define properly the assumed impact of gynaecological oncologists compared with other clinicians in the surgical management of ovarian cancer would necessitate a prospective randomised trial, and the practical and ethical obstacles involved make such a study improbable.

Debulking tumour is only one aspect of surgical intervention in ovarian cancer. Staging the disease correctly is important to facilitate management decisions. In this aspect of care who affords the best outcome? Many authors (Young *et al.* 1983; McGowan *et al.* 1985; Mayer *et al.* 1992) have reported that up to 20 per cent or more of patients with early-stage ovarian cancer will have their disease upstaged at a second laparotomy, often by disease detection within the relevant lymph nodes. However, is this a justification for the specialist over the generalist? First, one either considers appropriate staging important or irrelevant. There cannot be a selection process whereby those untrained in lymph node dissection disregard its importance, while the technically 'easier' staging processes are accepted. The presence of metastatic disease would affect adjuvant therapies. Whether or not survival of women with late-stage disease (by virtue of positive lymph nodes alone) is enhanced by adjuvant chemotherapy remains unknown. However, the consensus of medical/clinical oncologists' opinion would be to consider therapy for such women.

Puls *et al.* (1997) compared staging and chemotherapeutic management of a small group of patients (cared for by either a gynaecological oncologist or a general gynaecologist) and found that 6-year survival for early-stage disease was 90 per cent and 68 per cent respectively, with more patients in the former group receiving adjuvant chemotherapy. But such studies may only reflect the more careful selection process, in that correct staging identifies those patients with an inherent better survival. While this may be true, is it a sufficient challenge to present recommendations?

Few would disagree with the fact that doctors and *patients* are entitled to correct information regarding the disease stage, considering the implications regarding care and survival. With the knowledge that one in five inappropriately staged women with 'early' ovarian cancer will have a higher disease stage, there is an obligation to counsel patients honestly. Some may opt for further surgical intervention, and women are then exposed to an avoidable second operation, which carries a significantly higher morbidity than a primary procedure (Schueler *et al.* 1998). Although present information has gaps, this is not an excuse to ignore internationally agreed standards, and those opposing these should have firm justification for their stance.

The medical/clinical oncologist

Many women with ovarian cancer will receive adjuvant chemotherapy. Evidence relating specifically to any superior outcome if the medical/clinical oncologist has a particular subspecialist role in ovarian cancer is not available, although, as discussed above, circumstantial evidence does exist. Within these specialties, there would seem a natural evolution whereby individual oncologists care for specific cancer types, and interestingly this seems to be accepted rather than challenged. However, in some Nordic countries the gynaecological oncologist administers chemotherapy. Should this be considered in the UK? The main advantage would be in the continuity of patient care. Realistically, as there are few gynaecological oncologists, it is difficult to envisage how this would be achieved presently and also whether this would prove an advance in care.

The multidisciplinary team

There are many specialists who may become involved in caring for a woman with ovarian cancer. Survival is enhanced for women cared for by gynaecologists and within a multidisciplinary team setting, as derived from the report by Junor *et al.* (1994). Indeed, if all patients were cared for within such a setting, it is estimated that overall survival could be improved by up to 10 per cent. The study does not define the individual specialist's impact on outcome, nor the role of the gynaecological oncologist.

Cancer centres

Naturally, certain circumstances may exist whereby the patient, for a variety of reasons, requests care in the local hospital. Since the publication of the Calman/Hine report (Department of Health 1995) and the Royal College of Obstetricians and Gynaecologists' response (Kitchener 1997), many meetings have been held to discuss the centralisation of cancer services, including ovarian cancer. Such centres would have gynaecological and medical/clinical oncologists as part of the team.

A common objection to developing cancer centres is the stress and disruption caused to patients and their family and friends by the need to travel long distances to such hospitals, rather than to a local hospital. Admittedly, the isolation of the patient, and the accompanying stress is a real problem for some patients, and practically, it will be impossible to support innumerable centres. However, is this problem a sufficient challenge to the question posed or indeed does this concern accurately reflect the patient's desires? An interesting article from Canada (Feldman-Stewart *et al.* 1996) revealed that distance and family preoccupations were not at the forefront of cancer patients' concerns: most patients were more concerned about receiving accurate information on possible outcome and about the physician's skills.

Related to this is another Canadian study (Préfontaine & Gruslin 1995) assessing physicians' views on indications for referral of women with suspected ovarian cancer by a gynaecologist to a gynaecological oncologist. Although 87 per cent of respondents agreed that a patient's wishes were important in deciding referral, given the choice, 43 per cent of general gynaecologists would operate on women with obvious ovarian cancer and not refer to a gynaecological oncologist. This is of concern, as patients' views, though deemed important, have little impact on clinical decisions.

Conclusions

In the present era of evidence-based medicine, it is easy to challenge the perceived wisdom by insisting that changes should only be based on appropriately constructed prospective clinical studies. If this is accepted, then the *status quo* remains, which most probably means maintaining the present poor survival rates for this disease. Challenging this stance is the published information with all its inherent biases and limitations. This information does suggest that changing practice can potentially improve outcome. Can the perceived wisdom be truly challenged? Treating ovarian cancer in the context of surgical or medical care alone can give rise to a reasonable debate as to who performs best. Treating a woman with ovarian cancer adds an extra dimension to the debate: the care required involves many specialists. Who is most likely to have the structure to accommodate these multiple needs? Those within the multidisciplinary setting dealing regularly with ovarian cancer, with access to support services, and assessed by peers in order to ensure that the care provided conforms to the required standards – or those isolated and dealing with a small caseload of this rare cancer?

Challenging the perceived wisdom encourages careful consideration as to the best way to care for patients. The real challenge now is to deliver the best.

References

Boente M P, Chi D S & Hoskins W J (1998). The role of surgery in the management of ovarian cancer: primary and interval cytoreductive surgery. *Sem Oncol* **25**, 326–34.

Department of Health (1991). *Management of ovarian cancer: current clinical practice*. Standing Subcommittee on Cancer of the Ovary. DoH, London.

Department of Health (1995). *A policy framework for commissioning cancer services: a report by the Expert Advisory Group on Cancer to the Chief Medical Officers of England and Wales.* HM Stationery Office, London.

Eisenkop S M, Spiros N M, Montag T W, Nalick R H & Wang H J (1992). The impact of subspeciality training on the management of advanced ovarian cancer. *Gynecol Oncol* **47**, 203–9.

Feldman-Stewart D, Chammas S, Hayter C, Pater J & Mackillop W J (1996). An empirical approach to informed consent in ovarian cancer. *J Clin Epidemiol* **49**, 1259–69.

Junor EJ, Hole D J & Gillis C R (1994). Management of ovarian cancer: referral to a multidisciplinary team matters. *Brit J Cancer* **70**, 363–70.

Kehoe S (1996). Debulking surgery in ovarian cancer. *Brit J Obstet Gynaecol* **103**, 291–3.

Kehoe S, Powell J, Wilson S & Woodman C (1994). The influence of the operating surgeon's specialisation on patient survival in ovarian carcinoma. *Br J Cancer* **70**, 1014–17.

Kitchener H (1997). Gynaecological cancer services – time for a change. *Brit J Obstet Gynaecol* **104**, 123–6.

McGowan L, Lesher L P, Norris H J & Barnett M (1985). Mis-staging of ovarian cancer. *Obstet Gynecol* **65**, 568–72.

Mayer A R, Chambers S K, Graves E *et al.* (1992). Ovarian cancer staging: does it require a gynaecological oncologist? *Gynecol Oncol* **47**, 223–7.

Nguyen H N, Averette H E, Hoskins W, Penalver M, Sevin B U & Steren A (1993). National survey of ovarian carcinoma. Part V. The impact of physicians' specialty on patients' survival. *Cancer* **72**, 3663–70.

OPCS (1993). Mortality statistics. Series DH21, no.20. HMSO, London.

Pettersson F (1988). *Annual report of the results of treatment in gynecologic cancer.* International Federation of Gynaecology and Obstetrics (FIGO), vol.20.

Préfontaine M & Gruslin A (1995). Referral patterns for suspected ovarian cancer: a survey of practicing gynaecologists. *Int J Gynecol Cancer* **5**, 381–5.

Puls L E, Carrasco R, Morrow M S & Blackhurst D (1997). Stage I ovarian carcinoma: specialty-related differences in survival and management. *South Med J* **90**, 1097–100.

Roohan P J, Bickell N A, Baptiste M S, Therriault G D, Ferrara E P & Siu A L (1998). Hospital volume differences and five year survival from breast cancer. *Am J Public Health* **88**, 454–7.

Schueler J A, Trimbos J B, Hermans J & Fleurent G J (1998). The yield of surgical staging in presumed early stage ovarian cancer: benefits or doubts. *Int J Gynecol Cancer* **8**, 95–102.

Selby P, Gillis C & Haward R (1996). Benefits from specialised cancer care. *Lancet* **348**, 313–18.

Woodman C, Baghdady A, Collins S & Clyma J A (1997). What changes in the organisation of cancer services will improve the outcome for women with ovarian cancer. *Brit J Obstet Gynaecol* **104**, 135–9.

Young R C, Decker D G, Taylor Wharton J *et al.* (1983). Staging laparotomy in early ovarian cancer. *JAMA* **250**, 3072–6

Chapter 4

The pathway from early symptoms to referral

Wendy M N Reid

Introduction

The majority of women with ovarian cancer present with late-stage disease, with correspondingly poor outcomes. The management of ovarian cancer relies on the primary surgery accurately to stage the disease and proceed effectively allowing for the best results from chemotherapy. The Calman/Hine report (Department of Health 1995) has led to the development of cancer centres where the expertise and support mechanisms for the management of cancer will be concentrated. The literature supports the view that outcome is influenced by the place of surgery and the specialty training of the surgeon. The Scottish report *Fighting the silent killer* (Accounts Commission for Scotland 1997) addresses the difficulties in improving the outcome of ovarian cancer, but starts its management guidelines at when the diagnosis of the disease is suspected. If diagnosis is difficult then a primary referral along the pathway outlined in such guidelines may be impossible to achieve.

The nature of the symptoms from ovarian cancer means that presentation is often delayed or indeed the woman may be referred to another specialty or to a unit without a specialist interest in gynaecological cancer. The symptoms are vague and non-specific, including abdominal bloating and discomfort, pressure symptoms, such as urinary frequency, and nausea. Other gynaecological cancers have more specific presenting symptoms and signs, e.g. post-menopausal bleeding with endometrial cancer, an abnormal cervical smear with cervical cancer and vulval pruritus or a visible lesion with vulval cancer.

A review of the records

We reviewed the notes of 80 of the 108 cases of epithelial ovarian cancer identified from histopathology records and managed in our unit, from January 1991 to December 1997 inclusive. Eighteen sets of notes were unavailable as the patients were deceased and the notes had been microfilmed; there was, however, information on these cases from the pathology computer database. Ten sets of case notes were missing altogether. Ovarian cancer in our unit is managed by two named gynaecologists in conjunction with a third gynaecologist whose main interest is cervical and endometrial cancer and two medical oncologists who work with a team including palliative care, nursing and counselling health care professionals. For the purposes of this review we have considered 'appropriate referral' to be to one of this medical team.

First, we looked at the primary mode of referral. Sixty-six patients had been referred by a general practitioner to a variety of specialists: 28 to one or other of the recognised gynaecologists for this purpose, 18 to other gynaecology colleagues and 20 to other specialties. In 13 of the 66 referral letters, the word 'cancer' was mentioned; in 23 out of 66, the referral was marked 'urgent', and both 'cancer' and 'urgent' appeared in 11 letters. In 65 letters a diagnosis had been proposed, as shown in Table 4.1.

Table 4.1 Suggested diagnosis by referring GP

Diagnosis	No. of patients (n=66)
Pelvic mass	28
Prolapse	3
Fibroids	3
Pain	14
Others	17

Note: 'Others' include: menorrhagia, cystitis, hernia, claudication, appendicitis, backache, ascites, dyspepsia, dysphagia and post-menopausal bleeding

The 11 patients where the GP had mentioned both 'cancer' and 'urgent' had proposed diagnoses of a pelvic mass in seven cases; ascites, carcinomatosis and an abnormal smear in three other cases; and no diagnosis was made in one case. Of the 13 cases where the GP used the word 'cancer', nine women were referred with a pelvic mass; three, as previously stated, with ascites, carcinomatosis and an abnormal smear respectively; and one had no diagnosis made. The 23 women referred with letters using the word 'urgent' had a diagnosis of pelvic mass in 14 cases; two with pain and discomfort; and one each with ascites, carcinomatosis, dyspepsia, hernia, dysphagia, urinary retention and an abnormal smear.

The time from the date on the GP referral letter to the woman being seen in the gynaecology clinic was an average of 30.7 days. The range was from one day, following a telephone call to the gynaecologist, to 230 days; this woman had been referred with a femoral hernia as the main complaint and, when seen by the surgeons, was referred to the gynaecologists and seen three days later.

Eighteen women were referred to other gynaecologists and 34 to other specialties (see Table 4.2).

Table 4.2 Referrals to specialties other than gynaecology

Specialty	No. of patients (n=34)
Gastroenterology	9
General surgery	9
Accident & Emergency	14
Others	6

Note: 'Others' include: vascular surgery (1); neurology (1); oncology (1); endocrinology (1); psychiatry (1); and general medicine (1)

Fourteen cases were referred acutely to Accident & Emergency by GPs, six were seen and admitted by the general surgeons; five by the gynaecologists on call; one by neurology; one by gastroenterology; and one by the geriatricians.

In the 56 cases referred to other gynaecologists or other specialties, 43 diagnoses were suggested in the referral letter (see Table 4.3).

Table 4.3 Suggested diagnosis by referring GP to other gynaecologists/specialties

Diagnosis	No. of patients (n=43)
Pelvic mass	21
GI neoplasm	5
Diverticulitis	1
Irritable bowel syndrome	1
Hernia	2
Others	13

Note: 'Others' include: urinary retention, post-menopausal bleeding, fibroids, and bowel obstruction

Twenty-four cases were inpatients under the care of other specialties and then referred to the gynaecology or oncology team.

We looked at how other specialties had made the diagnosis of ovarian cancer or raised the suspicion of such a diagnosis. In 37 of the patients referred by other specialties, 33 had a pelvic ultrasound scan that led directly to the referral. In 17 of these 37 patients, a vaginal examination was performed, while 16 had a rectal examination. Twenty-three patients had tumour markers sent that included CA 125 and carcinoembryonic antigen (CEA) measurements. Eleven of the 37 had clinically detectable ascites. Other investigations performed included: chest X-ray; abdominal X-ray; intravenous urography; CT scan of abdomen & pelvis; barium enema; and sigmoidoscopy. In 11 of the 37 no pelvic examination was documented.

The time from referral by other specialties to being seen by the gynaecology team was 4.35 days on average. In 24 cases, the referral was made by junior trainees to other trainees or to the team and in 17 cases, by consultant colleagues to a named consultant gynaecologist.

The time from seeing the gynaecology team to having surgery was on average 21.5 days, with a range of 1 to 230 days. The patient who waited 230 days for surgery had been referred with prolapse and the ovarian mass was an incidental finding on admission – histology showed a borderline tumour.

The stage of disease at primary surgery was documented in 63 of the 80 case notes (see Table 4.4). These were all patients whose primary surgery was either performed by, or in the presence of, one of the recognised team. Of the 17 cases where no stage was documented, six were operated on by non-oncology trained gynaecologists, and 11 by other surgical specialties. Three of the cases operated on by other gynaecology colleagues were operated on acutely, and had no suspicious features noted at surgery. There were clinical signs of pelvic cancer at surgery in all of the 11 patients operated on by general surgeons, six of whom were acute cases.

Table 4.4 Stage at primary surgery

Stage	No. of patients
Stage I	15
Stage II	4
Stage III	33
Stage IV	11

Discussion

The data presented provide some evidence showing the difficulty we face as clinicians in making the diagnosis of ovarian cancer. Even in a unit where there are identifiable members of a team available to see such patients, the diagnosis can be delayed. Obviously, when the diagnosis is suspected, the fact that a dedicated team is available facilitates referral and allows appropriate treatment to be instituted rapidly.

The wide variety in choice of specialist for the primary referral reflects the diversity and vagueness of the disease symptomatology. The difficulties faced by general practitioners in accessing outpatient investigations, for example, may influence the referral, and we recognise that we do not have data on how many times a woman had presented to her GP with similar symptoms or how long her history had preceded referral.

The importance of the primary surgery, at the least providing accurate staging, is highlighted by the fact that of the women operated on approximately one in five were not staged at this time.

A suspected diagnosis of ovarian cancer should result in the woman being referred to the appropriate unit where accurate surgical staging and effective chemotherapy are available, in an environment that fosters good communication between health care professionals and the woman requiring treatment. There is, however, no evidence suggesting that the way in which women are referred has any influence on the outcome of treatment of this disease in terms of survival.

Delay at this stage, however, has other implications. A rapid diagnosis, effective, individualised surgery, and a collaborative approach from all involved result in efficient use of resources and in the woman and her family being accurately informed and supported at all stages of her treatment by a specialist team. Conversely, delay in referral can lead to increasing debility, particularly in the older patient.

The primary surgery may be inadequate and not provide the necessary information for adjuvant chemotherapy. Further surgery may be necessary, the patient may be confused as to the diagnosis and chemotherapy may be delayed. Many of these women will be managed as inpatients, or undergo extensive outpatient investigations, wasting resources and adding to the distress of the woman and her family when the diagnosis is finally reached. The ease of referral between specialties within the same hospital can be enhanced by good communication between consultant colleagues. A referral from one trainee doctor to another is less likely to result in appropriate, rapid assessment than if the referral is from consultant to consultant.

The Labour Government's White Paper *The new NHS* (Secretary of State for Health, 1997) states that 'all new patients with cancer will be seen by a specialist within two weeks'. This may be possible with adequate resources when a cancer has a clearly recognisable presentation, but seems unlikely to happen with ovarian cancer. As the greatest delay with this disease appears to occur between the primary referral and seeing the appropriate specialist, how can we improve our care? Obviously, if every woman with non-specific complaints such as abdominal bloating was to be referred for a consultant opinion, our outpatients' department would be overwhelmed. However, raising awareness both among women and among general practitioners that ovarian cancer is an insidious disease, with vague complaints and recognising the possibility that a few women will belong to one of the defined high-risk groups, may lead to women, and their family doctor, at least not ignoring the symptomatology.

Referrals from other specialties were mostly triggered by an abnormal pelvic ultrasound scan, and it may be that for a general practitioner this would be a reasonable test to consider. There is no recognised screening test as yet for the low-risk population, but an index of suspicion may create an environment where clinical examination and pelvic ultrasound will both have an enhanced role in making the diagnosis. Colleagues in other specialties need to be aware of the limitations of some investigations, and the importance of a full pelvic examination must be stressed. Gynaecologists involved in the management of ovarian cancer will also have to accept that a large proportion of the referrals will be for benign pelvic pathology and develop referral pathways that enable women to be seen rapidly. This should not add to the overall clinical workload as these are symptomatic patients rather than a screened population, but resources may need to be redistributed. The role of 'rapid access clinics' has yet to be evaluated in the pathway for diagnosing ovarian cancer, but may facilitate GP access to specialist investigations.

Conclusions

To define a referral pattern for a disease that presents with such vague symptoms is difficult, but the data we have presented show that raising awareness both among women and among health care professionals is necessary to allow early, appropriate referral. It remains to be seen whether this will impact on the survival rates for women with ovarian cancer.

Acknowledgements

The author is grateful to Kerstin Rolfe, Research Fellow (non-clinical), for collating the data presented, and other members of the Royal Free Ovarian Cancer Team: Prof. A B MacLean, Dr C Collis, Dr A Jones, Dr J Ledermann, Dr G Lieberman, Dr C Perrett, Dr A Slack and Dr A Tookman.

References

Accounts Commission for Scotland (1997). *Fighting the silent killer. Optimising the management of ovarian cancer in Scotland.* Accounts Commission for Scotland, Edinburgh

Department of Health (1995). *A policy framework for commissioning cancer services: a report by the Expert Advisory Group on Cancer to the Chief Medical Officers of England and Wales.* HM Stationery Office, London.

Secretary of State for Health (1997). *The new NHS.* Stationery Office, London (Cm 3807).

Chapter 5

Monitoring and follow-up of patients treated with chemotherapy for epithelial ovarian cancer

Chris J Poole & Digumarti Raghunadharao

Introduction

Epithelial ovarian cancer is an example of a solid tumour whose chemosensitivity can often provide the basis for good palliation and prolongation of life. The substitution of paclitaxel for cyclophosphamide, in combination with cisplatin, has been recently shown to improve the median survival of patients with newly diagnosed disease by 10–13 months (McGuire *et al.* 1996; Stuart *et al.* 1998). Furthermore, with the substitution of carboplatin for cisplatin, we have an easily administered standard regimen whose clinical benefits appear secure in the face of a low-grade denominator for treatment-related toxicity, and which is now, by consensus, standard treatment (Adams 1998; Neijt 1999; Ozols 1999).

However, the impact of paclitaxel's inclusion in first-line regimens on patients' long-term prospects may be less impressive (Sandercock *et al.* 1998). Certainly, the meagre 4-month prolongation of median progression-free survival forewarned of an ultimately limited effect in this respect (McGuire *et al.* 1993), and the substantive improvement in median survival reflects an asymmetric extension of second remission in patients who initially receive paclitaxel. Whether we see any improvement in the 5 per cent 10-year survival figure documented in long-term follow-up studies of patients treated with platinum-based chemotherapy in the mid-1980s remains to be seen (Warwick 1995). Even a proportional increase as large as 50 per cent would have but little absolute quantitative impact.

For many years, the main thrust of research into better treatment for ovarian cancer has been to discover drugs whose activity might better complement that of platinum. Although it is encouraging that the inclusion of drugs with relatively modest degrees of non-cross-resistance in first-line platinum combinations can have such worthwhile impact on medium-term survival, the persistent risk of recurrence has important implications for the direction of further work. First, it defines a need for studies designed to improve the management of relapse and reduce its morbidity; second, it prompts the urgent development of effective maintenance or consolidation strategies designed to prolong remission. Hitherto, neither of these areas has received much attention from clinical researchers. Both approaches might revolutionise the business of 'routine follow-up' as we know it, and put an end to the tradition of therapeutic passivity once the platinum bolt is shot.

This chapter will address the question of what might constitute optimal patient follow-up, given the limitations of the current evidence base (reviewed in Markman 1994). It will also review controversies about the management of relapse and discuss some more recent studies which explore the points of debate. Lastly, it will look at experimental consolidation and maintenance strategies.

Monitoring chemotherapy response

The follow-up of patients with ovarian cancer begins with monitoring their response and side-effects during chemotherapy. Recent studies of first-line cisplatin and paclitaxel (McGuire *et al.* 1996; Stuart *et al.* 1998) suggest that 75–77 per cent of patients' tumours will respond to treatment. The prompt identification of disease progression is important. The sooner can non-responding patients be identified by effective monitoring, the less toxicity will they suffer unnecessarily, the less money will be wasted on ineffective treatment and the sooner can consideration be given to more appropriate therapy. Depending on context, this might consist of simple symptomatic palliative care, early phase clinical trials, or off-study second-line 'salvage' chemotherapy. Although a counsel of excellence might demand routine pathology review for all patients with a diagnosis of ovarian cancer, UK health care resource issues render this impracticable as general policy before chemotherapy, and most clinicians would restrict expert pathology review to certain situations. These include tumours removed from younger patients, borderline histologies, and those morphologies (endometrioid and mucinous) which resemble metastases from gastrointestinal or other primary sites. However, review should arguably be standard practice in the face of a refractory response.

Monitoring response may be difficult. Traditional methods were primarily clinical, backed up by second-look laparotomy, as the ultimate arbiter. Typical symptomatic clues to an ongoing response comprise general constitutional improvement, reduction of abdominal bloating or swelling and resolution of pelvic symptoms such as urinary frequency or tenesmus. Reassuring findings on physical examination include diminution in the size of pelvic or abdominal masses, regression of palpable lymphadenopathy, and resolution of ascites or effusions. Second-look laparotomy fell from fashion as evidence amassed that secondary debulking, following completion of platinum-based chemotherapy, failed to impact on the subsequent natural history of the disease (Luesley *et al.* 1988). In these circumstances, surgical documentation of response seems increasingly unreasonable when presented as an end in itself, and it is now less frequently included in clinical trial protocols. However, the option of intervention debulking surgery is increasingly pursued, both on and off study, given provisional acceptance of its impact on survival and, secondarily, this allows the opportunity to gauge early pathological response (van der Burg *et al.* 1995).

Radiology is increasingly used to complement clinical assessment of response. At its simplest, a plain chest X-ray can confirm the resolution of a (cytologically positive) pleural effusion. However, for most patients radiological documentation of response means cross-sectional imaging. The preferred technique is pre- and post-chemotherapy computerised tomographic (CT) scans of the abdomen and pelvis. Unfortunately, routine CT scans remain outside the grasp of some UK clinicians, who may even have major problems in obtaining timely scans for the minority of patients treated in clinical trials. This difficulty has resulted in an increasing sensitivity to the obligatory use of interim scans in some protocols, and the impact this may have in exacerbating pressure on resources. While the excess costs of investigations in clinical trials are inevitably covered, the issue exorcising some ethics committees is their deleterious impact on unacceptably long waiting lists for routine scans.

The main technical limitation of CT scans is their failure to discriminate low-volume residual disease (Calkins *et al.* 1987; Bragg & Hricak 1993). However, while the literature suggests a trend towards magnetic resonance imaging (MRI) providing better definition of peritoneal tumour deposits (especially when there is ascites), there is consensus that any advantage may be marginal and outweighed by the greater costs and limited availability of MRI. The main strength of MRI lies with the contrast it provides between tumour and soft tissue (Scoutt & McCarthy 1991; Semelka *et al.* 1993; Kainz *et al.* 1994; Forstner *et al.* 1995). Ultrasound, which may be both cheap and quick, is operator-dependent, insensitive and non-specific (Murolo *et al.* 1989). This renders it totally unsuitable for independent review, in the context of monitoring response, and its use in clinical trials is therefore generally undesirable. Its utility is greatest in the initial investigation of a pelvic mass.

These problems and limitations have engendered considerable enthusiasm for the use of serological tumour markers as a means of monitoring response to chemotherapy (Rustin 1996; Rustin & Tuxen 1996). The availability of cheap high-quality commercial kits for CA 125 measurement, and their intuitively appreciated read-out, ensured their early popularity ahead of a hard evidence base (Rustin *et al.* 1992). The choice of CA 125 as the best available marker is beyond debate (Rustin *et al.* 1993). However, although more than 90 per cent of patients presenting with FIGO stage III or IV disease have an elevated CA 125 (Table 5.1), the proportion of patients with raised markers after surgery depends on the success of primary debulking (Table 5.2). An elevated CA 125 is more likely among those with serous and papillary tumour types, and less likely in those with endometrioid and mucinous morphologies, in whom measurement of carcino-embryonic agent (CEA) and CA 19.9 may sometimes be more useful (Table 5.3).

Table 5.1 CA 125 and stage at presentation

FIGO stage	% elevated (all histologies)	Mean CA 125 (U/ml)
Stage I	51	20
Stage II	71	20
Stage III	91	393
Stage IV	98	689

[*Source:* Markowska *et al.* 1990]

Table 5.2 CA 125 and tumour burden following primary debulking surgery

Post-operative residuum	n	% of patients with CA 125 >35 U/ml	Median CA 125 value (U/ml)
None	206	19	15
<2cm	46	54	43
2–5cm	74	78	104
>5cm	161	95	455

[*Source:* Makar *et al.* 1992a]

Table 5.3 CA 125 and histology

Histology	n	CA 125 (serum)	
		% > 35 U/ml	Median U/ml
Mixed	37	100	384
Serous	267	91	391
Unclassified	77	87	394
Clear cell	37	81	206
Endometrioid	43	70	199
Mucinous	20	55	49

[*Source:* Makar *et al.* 1992a]

While early work showed clear relationships between tumour burden after chemotherapy assessed at second-look laparotomy and pre-operative serum CA 125 (see Table 5.4), validation of CA 125 response criteria by formal comparison with objective clinical and radiological response data has been hampered by

33

difficulties in developing both robust and practical nomograms with which to describe and analyse CA 125 change in individual patients. For many, stringency and utility seemed impossible bedfellows. The requirements for a credible algorithm were formally defined by Rustin *et al.* (1996 a & b).

Table 5.4 CA 125 and tumour burden documented at second-look laparotomy

Residuum	n	% CA 125 >35 U/ml	Median CA 125 (U/ml)
PCR	50	2	8
Microscopic	23	4	10
<2cm	50	34	18
2-5cm	31	74	77
>5cm	54	94	330

[*Source:* Makar *et al.* 1992b]

He suggested they include the following:

- an inherent resemblance to standard response criteria;
- simplicity sufficient for routine clinical use;
- rigour sufficient for trials;
- sensitivity sufficient to apply to at least 50 per cent of patients;
- specificity sufficient for a false–positive prediction rate of less than 10 per cent.

In developing a nomogram, Rustin *et al.* considered several different approaches, using data from two North Thames Co-Operative Group chemotherapy trials (NT3 and NT4) as a test bed for their ideas. Some proposals proved immediately unsatisfactory; for example, any insistence on a normalisation of CA 125 tumour marker to score a response would clearly exclude some major falls and include some trivial reductions. Conversely, acceptance of any serial decrease in CA 125, without specified threshold percentage reduction was judged insufficiently precise. However, to discriminate a response conditional to a log fall in serum CA 125 would exclude all patients whose initial level was less than ten times normal.

It soon became clear that the use of a retrospectively acquired 'learning data set' was fraught with problems and would require the development of a cumbersome and complex model to include the majority of patients. To simplify matters, Rustin *et al.* took a pragmatic approach and cleaned up the learning data set itself. To be included, patients must have had a minimum of three CA 125 measurements made, with at least one CA 125 value $\geq$40 U/ml. The baseline reference CA 125 measurement must have been made either within 9 days prior to chemotherapy commencing, or within 35 days thereafter. Two trial populations were selected for the analysis, North Thames (NT) 3 and 4; on this basis, only 118/277 (43 per cent) of patients in NT3, and 186/254 (73 per cent) in NT4 had usable data.

Two sets of response criteria were then advanced. For either, any response must occur within 6 months of start of treatment. The '50 per cent response criteria' specified a minimum 50 per cent reduction in serum CA 125 across two measurements, and confirmed 28 days or more after the second. The '75 per cent response criteria' specified a serial fall in CA 125 of 75 per cent or more across three samples, subject to confirmation 28 days after response was first evident. The use of 'combined 50 per cent and 75 per cent criteria' provided response rates of 62 per cent in the NT3 trial and 55 per cent in NT4. It was felt these were on a par with response rates that might have been expected. However, no objective response rates were recorded in either trial. Rustin *et al.* looked to the Gynae Oncology Group (GOG) for corroborative data. GOG 97 was selected. It had accrued 451 patients, of whom 343 were evaluable for CA 125 response using Rustin criteria. However, only 107/343 had measurable disease by GOG criteria. Of these 107, 71 (66 per cent) had objective GOG responses. CA125 response sensitivity was 68 per cent in these. However, 14/34 recorded as stable by GOG were CA 125 responders. Hence, the overall CA 125 response rate was 66 per cent, identical to that recorded for conventional objective measures.

The use of the CA 125 tumour marker in phase II clinical trials has now also been examined, with similarly favourable results (Rustin *et al.* 1999).

A synthesis?

What then is the optimal approach to documentation of response? It is clear that the available techniques are on occasion individually unsatisfactory in terms of their applicability to all patients. However, do these shortcomings justify a 'belt and braces' approach to maximise the chances of documenting something? A counsel of excellence might well comprise the following: assessment of symptoms, performance status and clinical signs by medical staff before each cycle of chemotherapy is prescribed; CT scans of the abdomen and pelvis pre- and post-chemotherapy, with interim scans after two or three cycles; chest X-rays before and after the course, with interim films in the event of relevant abnormalities on the first and CA 125 marker measurement at baseline and after each cycle of chemotherapy.

However, can we customise this approach for the individual patient, to save expense, better use resources, reduce inconvenience, and improve safety? In all probability, we can, but the advantages would be modest. Certainly, the costs of these investigations pale into insignificance when compared with the costs of the newer drugs such as paclitaxel, topotecan, gemcitabine and docetaxel, and the financial waste implied by a non-responding patient receiving two or three more cycles of useless treatment in the face of early progression. We could reasonably dispense with serial tumour marker measurement in patients with marker-negative tumours, as defined by both pre-operative serological CA 125 values and tumour immunohistochemistry. Similarly, repeat CT scans would seem redundant in patients whose baseline films show no evidence of measurable or evaluable disease, and whose serial marker measurements and clinical assessments are in themselves reassuring. But what of patients with raised markers and measurable disease on CT scans? The available data suggest we could abandon scans outside the context of clinical trials, and simply adopt CA 125 measurements and clinical assessment. Anecdotally, a number of physicians have already adopted this as standard practice, particularly in palliative second- and third-line platinum-sensitive contexts. To take a more radical step, do we need CA 125 marker estimations repeated serially with each cycle of treatment? The evidence from one retrospective study (Redman *et al.* 1990) suggests that a 'limited sampling' methodology may predict an eventual response just as well. This requires prospective confirmation.

In the interim, should we continue to regard CT scans as necessary within trials? At present, the justifiably conservative consensus is yes. The risks of a wrong conclusion about the efficacy of a new drug and its potentially adverse impact on the management of many more patients are clearly unacceptable. More data about the validity of tumour marker response may change this view. However, many trial protocols continue to demand interim scans in patients with measurable disease. How much do these add to the management of patients with reassuring clinical findings and falling tumour marker trends? Arguably, it depends on the context. In phase II trials, interim scans may admittedly provide useful data about the rapidity of response, and its duration. 'Confirmation' scans, by convention undertaken one month after maximal response, are also frequently specified in early-phase studies. Their justification is their pivotal importance in properly documenting beyond all reasonable doubt a relatively small number of events which may have major implications for the appropriate direction of subsequent resource- and patient-hungry larger studies.

By contrast, such detailed investigations as interim scans in the phase III setting arguably amount to waste of resources. Not only does the vast majority of previously untreated patients given chemotherapy for newly diagnosed ovarian cancer have either an objective or stable response, but the primary endpoints should relate more closely to clinical utility, and comprise measurement of progression-free survival, median survival, and overall survival at specified time points. Complete and partial response rates are usually defined as secondary endpoints in large phase III studies and one pre- and post-treatment CT scan could suffice for their documentation. The judicious use of interim scans could be reserved for those patients with rising tumour markers or clinical indication of non-response. The difficulties implicit in measuring progression-free survival, and interpreting overall survival figures will be addressed later.

Unfortunately, for some UK oncologists these sophisticated arguments are an arcane irrelevance. However, the scandalous difficulty they face in arranging prompt routine scans is not a simple cost issue. At about £200, a CT scan is cheap. The problem is the limited availability of the resource, the 'CT slot', and the lack of managerial vision implied by allowing an expensive item of capital like a CT scanner to cool down at night. In Hyderbad, India, CT scanners are run round the clock, and there are no waiting lists.

Monitoring chemotherapy toxicity

Side-effects are an inevitable consequence of cytotoxic usage. Their precise nature varies from drug to drug. Genetic susceptibility aside, their frequency in a population and individual severity relate to the dose intensity and schedule used. Pharmacokinetic parameters such as 'AUC' (area under concentration/time curve), or time above some threshold concentration value may be more accurate predictors of toxicity for some drugs. For others total cumulative dose is better. Although the emphasis of latter-day care is increasingly prediction of risk in individual patients, careful monitoring remains necessary to detect unusual sensitivities and seize every opportunity to moderate their severity. Underlying medical conditions, performance status, renal and hepatic function are usually important in formulating this risk, and defining the pattern of monitoring necessary.

Chemotherapy side-effects are commonly classed as acute and reversible, or chronic and irreversible. Acute toxicities such as myelosuppression and oral mucositis typically represent the impact of chemotherapy on susceptible normal cell populations whose physiological state is one of rapid proliferation. Dose–response relationships for acute toxicity are usually steep. The proliferative response of stem cells in repopulating a denuded compartment provides for recovery. Their resilience is probably a function of their physiological redundancy: the majority of stem cells are in a resting phase of the cell cycle (G_0) at any one time and therefore kinetically resistant to chemotherapy's effects. Cumulative marrow toxicity – progressive slowing of marrow recovery across successive courses of chemotherapy – probably reflects attrition of stem cell reserves.

From the point of view of ovarian cancer chemotherapy, the most significant improvements in treatment-related toxicity have followed the introduction of carboplatin, which is largely free of the cumulative nephrotoxic and neurotoxic effects of cisplatin, as well as being considerably less emetogenic. Carboplatin's dose-limiting toxicity is myelosuppression and its usual reversibility is euphemistically claimed to be 'manageable'. Carboplatin also has the advantage of a simple pharmacokinetic disposition. Most is renally cleared unchanged and there is no significant metabolism. This permits optimisation of individual patient dose using pharmacokinetic principles, based on desired carboplatin concentration/time profile (AUC) (Calvert *et al.* 1989). This approach to dosing thus minimises significant interpatient variation in myelosuppression, and with it the hazards of thrombocytopenic haemorrhage and neutropenic sepsis. In this respect the action has moved from passive monitoring of side-effects to prediction and monitoring of renal function.

The more recent introduction of paclitaxel has brought problems of its own. These include acute hypersensitivity reactions, occasionally troublesome musculoskeletal aches and pains, and peripheral neuropathies. However, its myelosuppressive effects are short and brief, and rarely contribute to risks of sepsis. Furthermore, it may moderate the thrombocytopenic effects of carboplatin. The risk of acute hypersensitivity reactions necessitates the routine use of antihistamine and high-dose steroid premedication, but despite this precaution about 4 per cent of patients may be expected to encounter severe acute reactions, requiring further intervention. The basis for this vulnerability is idiosyncratic, and unknown. Risks seem maximal in the first few minutes of first and second infusions, and patients therefore require careful observation by trained nursing staff at this time. The probability of developing severe disabling peripheral neuropathy seems greatest in those with concomitant medical conditions which themselves involve the peripheral nerves, such as diabetes and alcoholism, or those previously exposed to neurotoxic agents such as cisplatin. However, careful monitoring is essential in all patients, as unexplained sensitivities do arise, and their rate of onset can, on occasion, surprise. Proprioceptive and 128 Hz vibration sense impairment are probably the most vulnerable modalities and therefore the most sensitive for monitoring purposes.

Unfortunately, many of the problems suffered by patients during chemotherapy have their origins in obligatory polypharmacy and side-effects which do not originate in the cytotoxic *per se*, but rather as a result of drugs prescribed to moderate chemotherapy effects. Some are particularly difficult to recognise as they may manifest as disease-related problems, or even exacerbations of the problem they were intended to deal with. Examples include dexamethasone, an essential component of antiemetic prophylaxis, which can itself cause dyspepsia and heartburn, and ostensibly exacerbate vomiting, and which frequently requires treatment with concomitant H2 antagonists or proton pump inhibitors. Metoclopromide-induced akathisia (restlessness) is a *forme-fruste* of dystonia which often resembles or exacerbates hospital phobia or panic attacks. Similarly, the 5HT-3 antagonists may cause constipation so severe as to be complicated by abdominal colic and vomiting, with physical signs and radiological features of bowel obstruction. This may be particularly difficult to manage in the context of high-volume peritoneal disease and visceral involvement, and a case can be made for the routine prophylactic use of aperients and glycerine suppositories.

Follow-up

Follow-up is unfashionable. Its contribution to the effective management of ovarian cancer is unproven. When put on the defensive by iconoclasts, clinicians' usual riposte is that it provides patients with reassurance and that patients like it. However, for many patients, the gritty reality is that follow-up may prove both time-consuming and stressful; it usually involves 'degrading' pelvic examinations, the 'tyranny' of CA 125 measurement, and potentially unsettling exposure to other patients who may not be doing so well. However, for the anxious, the overall balance seems positive. Even patients who are themselves health care professionals, with considerable insight into the limitations of the process, may say 'I'd be OK if I could come every fortnight'. Is this 'addiction to the clinic'? Not in all cases. Concerns about 'what will happen after chemotherapy has finished' are common from its start. However, a number of patients seem to reach their point of maximum anxiety between being told their immediate post-chemotherapy investigations have confirmed complete remission and while waiting for their next outpatient appointment two or three months later. Having been supported for five months by the close-range ministrations of the multidisciplinary team, they often feel suddenly 'cast adrift', and less able to face the vagaries of fate than they were the discomfort of regular chemotherapy. Studies that address patient preference, and scrutinise the subjective psychological benefit of different approaches are long overdue. There even seems scope for adjusting frequency of follow-up to the measured anxiety level of the patient.

Although hard evidence of clinical benefit in standard practice is lacking, what is obvious is that some form of follow-up is required to define endpoints of clinical trials. In particular, it is an absolute requirement for the development of new consolidation or maintenance strategies in first or second remission, and a number of these proposals will be discussed later. However, properly conducted follow-up studies, in particular those using multivariate analytical techniques, have on occasion provided valuable insights into the natural history of this disease.

Follow-up studies

Two sets of follow-up studies have been particularly pivotal in developing different aspects of everyday clinic treatment policy. The first defined those groups of patients more likely to benefit from platinum-containing second-line chemotherapy; the second has helped ensure the effective evaluation of adjuvant therapy in early-stage disease. By contrast, studies posing systematic questions about follow-up itself are few, and rather more recent. The rationale of follow-up in many malignant conditions is predicated on the notion that early diagnosis of relapse may improve prognosis. A trial to test this assumption in ovarian cancer has only recently commenced.

Follow-up studies which have used multivariate analysis to determine those factors predictive of response to second-line platinum-based chemotherapy have had a major influence on the pattern of use of chemotherapy at relapse. The first, and arguably most influential, was published by George Blackledge in 1989 (see Table 5.5). This analysed 93 patients' responses to platinum-containing phase II (second-line) regimens and showed that FIGO stage at presentation and time elapsed since completion of first-line therapy were the major predictors of response. Confirmatory data were presented by Gore *et al.* in 1990, and Markman in 1991. These studies have led to the near-universal adoption of treatment conventions which limit the evaluation of drugs in early-phase clinical trials to those patients relapsing within 6–12 months of completing first-line platinum-based chemotherapy. For patients relapsing after this time, these studies suggested the balance of advantage lay in favour of platinum re-exposure.

Table 5.5 Determinants of response to second-line platinum-based combination chemotherapy

Interval (months)	Total No.	No. responding	% response
<6	50	5	10
7–12	17	5	30
13–18	17	16	94

[*Source:* Blackledge *et al.* 1989]

These studies have also helped resolve more recent paradoxes. One of the ostensibly inexplicable findings of the GOG 111 trial concerned how a four-month difference in median progression-free survival (in favour of paclitaxel and cisplatin) might have hardened into a more substantive 13-month difference in median survival. The implication of this finding was paradoxical: the type of first-line therapy allocated could determine not just the duration of first remission, but also impact on length of second remission too. Furthermore, prolongation of second remission seemed disproportionate, in relation to the modest effect on the first. This finding had no immediately obvious precedent, and no easy explanation. It was one of several factors which delayed the adoption of paclitaxel and platinum as standard first-line therapy in the UK, and prompted the ICON-3 trial.

In GOG 111, most patients in both arms were re-exposed to a platinum regimen at relapse, and only a minority received second-line paclitaxel. Did the inclusion of paclitaxel in first-line regimens (and by implication perhaps a response to paclitaxel) somehow sensitise patients to subsequent platinum salvage? What could explain this effect? However, as data from the EORTC/Canadian-NCI/Scottish OV10 Intergroup study matured, a similar effect became clear, and OV10 differed from GOG 111 in respect of a higher proportion of patients receiving paclitaxel second line.

Other candidate explanations were advanced. Might paclitaxel exaggerate the Gompertzian qualities of ovarian cancer's growth curve, and have a disproportionate effect in retarding growth of larger tumours more than microscopic disease? Such an effect might plausibly result from the drug's anti-angiogenic qualities, blood vessel growth being required for macroscopic tumour progression.

However, with hindsight, the explanation may be simpler than any of the above. We know that the prospects of response to platinum rechallenge depend on duration of first remission, and that we might therefore anticipate modest differences in the inherent platinum sensitivity of populations of patients relapsing at medians of 14 months and 18 months. Plausibly, such differences in drug sensitivity could influence survival. We know responders generally live longer. This hypothesis could be tested using GOG 111, OV10 and ICON-3 data sets, by examining the relationships between progression-free survival and median survival in different groups of patients treated on their control arms. We would predict that a group of controls whose median progression-free survival was 18 months would have a median survival of 36 months.

Another example of a follow-up study which has made a major contribution to our understanding of the natural history of ovarian cancer was begun at the Royal Marsden Hospital in 1980 (Ahmed et al. 1996). It was a simple design, which prospectively logged all women presenting with surgically treated stage I invasive disease between 1980 and 1994. No patient received adjuvant chemotherapy. Patients were seen every three months for two years for symptomatic assessment, physical examination and measurement of serum CA 125. During this period, CT scans were undertaken every six months. Between two and five years after diagnosis, patients were seen six-monthly for examination and CA 125, and CT scans were done annually. In years 5–10, patients underwent annual physical examination and serum CA 125; CT scans were undertaken only if clinically indicated.

The study enrolled 194 patients and used multivariate analysis to define factors predictive of relapse. With a median follow-up of 54 months (range 7–157 months), tumour grade, the presence of ascites (even without cytological data) and surface tumour were independent poor prognostic factors for recurrence. Neither FIGO substage nor intra-operative rupture proved significant in this respect. None of these factors, at the time of analysis, had significant impact on survival.

Five-year survival for stage Ia was 94 per cent; stage Ib 92 per cent; and stage Ic 84 per cent. The study recommended that patients presenting with either stage Ia/b with high-grade histology, or stage Ic by virtue of pre-operative rupture or capsular involvement, be considered for adjuvant chemotherapy trials. All other patients were judged to have too low a risk of relapse to justify trials of adjuvant chemotherapy.

The response rate of 50 patients to salvage therapy at relapse in Wilshaw's study was just 44 per cent, perhaps a little lower than might be ordinarily expected in first-line chemotherapy. This is interesting in the context of Blackledge's second-line data. Here early stage at presentation (and by inference relapse after adjuvant therapy, rather than therapy for advanced disease) was an independent predictor for response.

Follow-up for patients treated outside trials

The hard fact remains that despite Department of Health advice, only a small minority of patients will be offered the chance to take part in clinical trials, or bask in someone's academic interest in their disease. Given the dearth of objective evidence about its psychological benefits or shortcomings, can follow-up be justified on other grounds? Many would regard its primary purpose as the detection and management of relapse. Do we any have evidence that follow-up and the way it is undertaken can significantly impact on outcome of relapse? Can we detect relapse 'early' and if we can, is prompt intervention advantageous?

The early detection of relapse

CA 125 marker studies have shown that a rising CA 125 tumour marker is both a sensitive and specific indicator of relapse. Rustin undertook the pivotal study, which has defined progression of ovarian cancer using CA 125 rise (Rustin *et al.* 1996 a & b). Using a 255-patient North Thames study addressing treatment duration, Rustin chose a CA 125 value of 30 U/ml as the upper limit of normal, and found that a doubling in value of CA 125 to 60 U/ml or more would define progression with a sensitivity of 85.9 per cent, and specificity of 91.3 per cent, in relation to standard techniques. The positive predictive value was 94.8 per cent, and the negative predictive value was 77.8 per cent.

Furthermore, several studies have shown that regular measurement of CA 125 provides a median of between 4 and 9 months' advance warning of clinically occult relapse, with a range from 1 to 24 months. Data from some of these studies are shown in Table 5.6.

Most chemotherapy trials now specify follow-up visit interval, frequency of CA 125 measurement, and precise indication for CT scans. The place of regular cross-sectional imaging in routine follow-up is unclear. Early work suggested little benefit. Results rarely seemed to affect management (Gore *et al.* 1989). However, scans during follow-up may have considerable utility in defining the point of progression.

Table 5.6 Tumour markers in the management of patients with ovarian cancer

CA 125 lead time on clinical relapse

Author	+ve lead time	Range (m)	Median (m)
Fisken (1990)	14/20	2–14.8	8.6
Ward (1993)	10/20	1–24	6.6
Hising (1991)	12/29	1–10	3
Niloff (1986)	3/35	NA	3
Bruzzone (1990)	17/41	1–9	NA
Gard (1994)	41/57	1–12	3.8
			Total 62%

[*Source:* Tuxen *et al.* 1995]

This is an increasingly important endpoint in phase III studies because of the wider availability of second-line salvage regimens, which may have confounding effects on any emerging survival difference attributable to the introduction of novel agents in first line. However, their utility in this setting is predicated on their use being incorporated into a protocol, and applied with equal frequency in both arms. If left to clinicians' discretion, prejudice about the likely outcome of a study might lead to their asymmetric imposition, with more frequent scans in control-arm patients, for example. Such bias could be ultimately self-fulfilling, and exaggerate the significance of what might otherwise have been a modest difference in progression-free interval. The most economic and sensible approach is to undertake a scan in response to a confirmed doubling of the CA 125 marker, or to investigate clinical abnormality, whether symptom or physical sign. CA 125 negative tumours may merit routine interval scans, on study. CEA and CA 19.9 markers may also be useful, particularly in CA 125 negative tumours.

Early intervention at relapse

Patients' views about this issue may be clearer than those of their doctors. The universal impact of stage, tumour burden, performance status and their surrogates on prognosis has entered the collective consciousness of the nation, and the majority of patients make the assumption that the purpose of follow-up is the early identification of relapse. Undoubtedly, the view that this matters is often reinforced by the considerable difficulties many patients will have suffered in obtaining prompt initial diagnosis, and most will have made the assumption that it was the delays therein which led them to require chemotherapy in the first place.

Close regular follow-up certainly affords the facility for early recognition of relapse, but does this benefit patients by reducing either the morbidity of their disease or subsequent treatment, or by improving quality of life or survival? We lack the data to know. However, these are extremely important questions and, for once, there are some well-designed trials under way to address them.

The management of relapse

There are two schools of thought about this. One, widely held in the UK, takes the view that as second-line therapy is never curative, it should properly be regarded as palliative. Palliation means symptom control and as chemotherapy has nasty side-effects, treatment ahead of symptoms can only be a nonsense. This view holds that it is therefore good practice to delay intervention until their advent. This approach is in keeping with conservative instincts, and ostensibly consoled by data from Blackledge (1989), which showed the longer the platinum-free interval, the higher the prospects of response to second-line chemotherapy.

The other view contradicts this point by point. It has greater currency in North America. Consonant with the central dogma of prognostic oncology, that tumour burden and performance status are all, it proposes that the earlier patients are treated at relapse the better. There are data to suggest that increased tumour volume has an adverse effect: prospects of response are lower for patients with measurable disease greater than 5 cm in diameter, for example (Eisenhauer *et al.* 1997). Furthermore, common experience suggests that bowel obstruction may sometimes occur as the first manifestation of relapse. Obstruction is at best a debilitating event with cataclysmic impact on treatment-related morbidity, and costs of care. At worst, it is a terminal event. Many would take the view that in the absence of a potential surgical solution, its advent would indicate that the time for cytoreductive intervention is past, and the opportunity lost. Hence to cite the Blackledge data in support of a conservative stance is to be guilty of gross over-extrapolation. Some North American trained clinicians would add to this that patients in the USA are by nature less likely to accept a conservative 'lets watch and wait' approach, and would feel that such nihilism simply reflected the poverty of 'socialist medicine' across the North Atlantic, an analysis which would culminate in unfavourable reference to UK survival figures for ovarian cancer.

What became clear in the early 1990s, was that only in Europe could we address the question of optimal timing of chemotherapeutic intervention in relapse in a prospective randomised trial. After several groups had grappled with unsuccessful designs and failed, Rustin produced the first feasible proposal and his protocol subsequently secured support from the Medical Research Council (MRC).

The design of MRC OVO5 is predicated on the early warning of radiological or clinical relapse afforded by regular CA 125 tumour marker measurement. Patients are registered once they have achieved radiological and marker remission following induction chemotherapy, and followed up 3-monthly with clinical assessment and CA 125 measurement. Key to the study's feasibility was the proposal that CA 125 data be made available only to the clinical trials office in the first instance. In the event of a significant rise, the trial co-ordinator randomises the patient to either inform the responsible clinician, with a view to commencing immediate chemotherapy, or not inform the clinician, in which case intervention would be deferred until clinically indicated. After a confirmatory marker measurement, the chemotherapy chosen is left to the consultant's discretion.

At the time of writing, 250 patients have been registered by the MRC, in a little over two years. However, the EORTC have recently launched the same protocol (EORTC 55955) and joint analysis is planned. A maximum of 1,100 patients will be registered, for up to 800 randomisations. Eighteen UK centres and three overseas centres are taking part in the MRC study.

The role of surgery at relapse

Kehoe, in Birmingham, has recently launched a randomised trial, the REACT study (Relapsed Ovarian Carcinoma and Cytoreductive Surgery Trial) to evaluate the role of surgery in patients relapsing 12 months or more from completion of first-line platinum-based chemotherapy. This study will need 300 patients in each arm, and clearly require national collaboration. The EORTC are exploring an intervention debulking study in the same clinical context.

Consolidation and maintenance therapies

The high relapse rate of patients treated with platinum-based chemotherapy for epithelial ovarian cancer, estimated at 90 per cent in some long-term follow-up studies, provides the rationale for trials of maintenance and consolidation therapy (Vermorken 1994). However, there remain basic uncertainties about the optimal duration of first-line therapy, relating to the limited power of the small number of studies addressing this question. Furthermore, all were completed in the 'pre-Taxol era' (Bertelsen *et al.* 1999). Hitherto, enthusiasm for consolidation studies has been bridled by the modest non-cross-resistant activity of the available drugs, and concerns about the debilitating nature of protracted treatment regimens, particularly in more elderly patients: sequential chemotherapy regimens utilising cisplatin and paclitaxel documented cumulative neurological toxicity as problematic (Poole *et al.* 1997). Other studies in this setting therefore employed either systemic dose intensification approaches, or locoregional chemotherapy using the peritoneal compartment. Renewed interest in a sequential approach to treatment has been partly engendered by discussion of the results of GOG 132 (Muggia 1997): in the cisplatin 'only' arm of this trial, a significant proportion of patients evidently were crossed over to paclitaxel ahead of disease progression, prompting many to attribute the relative success of this arm to this eventuality. The GOG and MRC are currently considering trial designs which formally test 'sequential couplets', and treatment duration questions, as candidates for inclusion in the next round of randomised phase III trials.

SWOG have already commenced a paclitaxel maintenance trial, prompted by data suggesting that paclitaxel-induced stabilisation of disease may have greater impact in the natural history of ovarian cancer than inspection of objective response rates may sometimes suggest (Markman *et al.* 1994).

Some of the more interesting maintenance and consolidation studies have explored the use of biological host response modifiers, such as alpha interferon, and targeted therapies, such as matrix metalloproteinase inhibitors, in the hope of avoiding the cumulative toxic effects of chemotherapy. The Yorkshire interferon study is one such trial. This took patients with complete or partial remissions following platinum-based chemotherapy and randomised them to alpha interferon 4.5 mega units, injected subcutaneously, thrice weekly, for up to two years, vs. standard follow-up. Patients were seen for two-monthly physical examination and CA 125 measurement with six-monthly CT scans for the first two years, and followed up three-monthly thereafter. Quality of life data were also gathered. Accrual was slow. The trial opened in 1990, and closed in 1997, with 300 patients randomised. Analysis is expected in July 1999. Arguably its modest size will render it underpowered to detect an intuitively likely level of benefit.

Matrix metalloproteinase inhibitors have, as yet, had an even unhappier evaluation. Matrix metalloproteinases (MMPs) are a homologous family of enzymes that are involved in tissue remodelling and morphogenesis. The extracellular matrix is the principal barrier to tumour growth and spread, and there is increasing evidence that their MMP expression may contribute to invasive, metastatic and angiogenic aspects of the malignant phenotype (Brown 1995). Inhibitors of MMP function therefore represent an attractive new class of targeted anticancer agents (Rasmussen & McCann 1997). Several have been shown to inhibit the spread and growth of a number of malignant tumours in animal models. Batimastat (BB94) was the first to enter clinical trial, but had poor oral bioavailability, and the occurrence of severe abdominal pain when delivered intraperitoneally prompted a halt to its development. Marimastat (BB2516), with good oral bioavailability and potent broad-spectrum activity against a number of MMPs, entered disease-specific phase I dose-ranging studies in 1994/5 (Poole *et al.* 1996; Nemunaitis *et al.* 1998). A variety of musculoskeletal problems were identified as dose-limiting toxicities. Marimastat is now the subject of randomised trials in several different solid tumours, and therapeutic contexts. Among the most important of these are maintenance studies. Unfortunately, a double-blind, placebo-controlled, randomised trial of maintenance marimastat, conducted in patients who had responded to second-line carboplatin, has recently been closed prematurely by the sponsor, British Biotech. The reasons for this remain unclear. Poor recruitment was cited, but this was an ostensibly specious argument since the same investigators were also actively recruiting to a parallel Biotech study addressing concurrent carboplatin and marimastat in the second-line context, and patients who entered this study were naturally excluded. Maintenance studies could not therefore be expected to recruit from the same investigator base, until the 'upstream' studies were closed. More significantly, perhaps, the FDA has recently shown reluctance to accept time to progression advantage as the basis for successful licence applications, and expressed the view that data which demonstrated survival, or quality of life advantage were preferred. This has important, as yet unresolved, implications for the design of maintenance studies in general. Time to progression was chosen as the primary endpoint for the Biotech marimastat maintenance trial as it provided the cleanest and most informative scientific output, free of the potentially confounding influence that subsequent third-line cytoreductive treatment might have on survival, for example. A larger and more adequately designed Bayer maintenance study continues, with the MMP inhibitor and antiangiogenic compound Bay-12-9566. Agouron Pharmaceuticals also have an MMP inhibitor (AG 3340) in phase III trials, with chemotherapy in other solid tumours. Watch this space.

References

Adams M, Calvert A H *et al*. (1998). Chemotherapy for ovarian cancer – a consensus statement on standard practice. (Editorial) (see comments). *Br J Cancer* **78**(11), 1404–6.

Ahmed F Y, Wiltshaw E, A'Hern R P, Nicol B, Shepherd J, Black P, Fisher C & Gore M E (1996). Natural history and prognosis of untreated stage I epithelial ovarian cancer. *J Clin Oncol* **14**, 2968–75.

Bertelsen K, Grenman S *et al*. (1999). How long should first-line chemotherapy continue? *Ann Oncol* **10**(Suppl.1), 17–20.

Blackledge G, Lawton F *et al*. (1989). Response of patients in phase II studies of chemotherapy in ovarian cancer: implications for patient treatment and design of phase II trials. *British Journal of Cancer* **59**(4), 650–3.

Bragg D G & Hricak H (1993). Imaging in gynecologic malignancies. *Cancer* **71**(Suppl.4), 1648–51.

Brown P D (1995). Matrix metalloproteinase inhibitors: a novel class of anticancer agents. *Adv Enzyme Regul* **35**, 293–301.

Calkins A R, Stehman F B *et al.* (1987). Pitfalls in interpretation of computed tomography prior to second-look laparotomy in patients with ovarian cancer. *Br J Radiol* **60**(718), 975–9.

Calvert A H, Newell D R, Gumbrell L A *et al.* (1989). Carboplatin dosage: prospective evaluation of a simple formula based on renal function. *J Clin Oncol* **17**(11), 1748–56.

Eisenhauer E A, Vermorken J B & van Glabbeke M (1997). Predictors of response to subsequent chemotherapy in platinum-pretreated ovarian cancer: a multivariate analysis of 704 patients. *Annals of Oncology* **8**, 963–8.

Forstner R, Hricak H *et al.* (1995). Ovarian cancer: staging with CT and MR imaging. *Radiology* **197**(3), 619–26.

Gore M E, Cooke J C, Wiltshaw E, Crow J M, Cosgrove D O & Parsons C S (1989). The impact of computed tomography and ultrasonography on the management of patients with carcinoma of the ovary. *Br J Cancer* **60**, 751–4.

Kainz C, Prayer L *et al.* (1994). The diagnostic value of magnetic resonance imaging for the detection of tumor recurrence in patients with carcinoma of the ovaries. *J Am Coll Surg* **178**(3), 239–44.

Luesley D, Lawton F *et al.* (1988). Failure of second-look laparotomy to influence survival in epithelial ovarian cancer. *Lancet* **2**(8611), 599–603.

Makar A P, Kristensen G B, Kaern J, Bormer O P, Abeler V M & Trope C G (1992a). Prognostic value of pre- and post-operative serum CA 125 levels in ovarian cancer. New aspects and multivariate analysis. *Obstet Gynecol* **79**(6), 1002–10.

Makar A P, Kristensen G B, Bormer O P & Trope C G (1992b). CA 125 measured before second-look laparotomy is an independent prognostic factor for survival in patients with epithelial ovarian cancer. *Gynecol Oncol* **45**(3), 323–8.

Markman M (1994). Follow-up of the asymptomatic patient with ovarian cancer. *Gynecol Oncol* **55**, S134–7.

Markman M, Hakes T, Barakt R, Curtin J, Almadrones L & Hoskins W (1996). Follow-up of Memorial Sloan-Kettering Cancer Centre patients on NCI protocol 9103. *J Clin Oncol* **14**, 796–9.

Markowska J, Kojczynski Z, Szewierski Z & Manys G (1990). CA 125 in monitoring chemotherapy of patients with ovarian cancer. *E J Gynaecol Oncol* **11**(3), 209–14.

McGuire W, Hoskins W *et al.* (1993). A phase III trial comparing cisplatin/cytoxan and cisplatin/taxol in advanced ovarian cancer. American Society of Clinical Oncology, Orlando, Fl.

McGuire W, Hoskins W *et al.* (1996). Cyclophosphamide and cisplatin compared with paclitaxel and cisplatin in patients with stage III and stage IV ovarian cancer. *New England Journal of Medicine* **334**, 1–6.

Muggia F, Braly P *et al.* (1997). Phase III trial of cisplatin or paclitaxel versus their combination in sub-optimal stage III and IV epithelial ovarian cancer: GOG study132. *ASCO Proceedings* **16**, 352a.

Murolo C, Costantini S *et al.* (1989). Ultrasound examination in ovarian cancer patients. A comparison with second look laparotomy. *J Ultrasound Med* **8**(8), 441–3.

48

Neijt J P & du Bois A (1999). Paclitaxel/carboplatin for the initial treatment of advanced ovarian cancer. *Semin Oncol* **26**(1)(Suppl.2), 78–83.

Nemunaitis J, Poole C *et al.* (1998). Combined analysis of studies of the effects of the matrix metalloproteinase inhibitor marimastat on serum tumor markers in advanced cancer: selection of a biologically active and tolerable dose for longer-term studies. *Clin Cancer Res* **4**(5), 1101–9.

Ozols R (1999). *ASCO Proceedings* 18.

Poole C, Adams M *et al.* (1996). A dose-finding study of marimastat, an oral matrix metalloproteinase-inhibitor in patients with advanced ovarian cancer. *Annals of Oncology* **7**, 68.

Poole C, Perren T *et al.* (1997). Sequential paclitaxel and cisplatin chemotherapy in patients with newly diagnosed epithelial ovarian cancer. *ASCO Proceedings* **16**, 356a.

Rasmussen H S & McCann P P (1997). Matrix metalloproteinase inhibition as a novel anticancer strategy: a review with special focus on batimastat and marimastat. *Pharmacol Ther* **75**(1), 69–75.

Redman C W, Blackledge G R, Kelly K, Powell J, Buxton E J & Luesley D M (1990). Early serum CA 125 response and outcome in epithelial ovarian cancer. *Eur J Cancer* **26**(5), S93–6.

Rustin G J (1996). Circulating tumor markers in gynecological tumors. *Curr Opin Oncol* **8**(5), 426–31.

Rustin G & Tuxen M (1996). Use of CA 125 in follow-up of ovarian cancer. (Letter). *Lancet* **348**(9021), 191–2.

Rustin G J, van der Burg M E *et al.* (1993). Advanced ovarian cancer. Tumour markers. *Ann Oncol* **4**(Suppl.4), 71–7.

Rustin G J, Nelstrop A *et al.* (1992). Savings obtained by CA-125 measurements during therapy for ovarian carcinoma. The North Thames Ovary Group. *Eur J Cancer* **28**(1), 79–82.

Rustin G J, Nelstrop A E *et al.* (1996a). Defining response of ovarian carcinoma to initial chemotherapy according to serum CA 125. *J Clin Oncol* **14**(5), 1545–51.

Rustin G J, Nelstrop A E *et al.* (1996b). Defining progression of ovarian carcinoma during follow-up according to CA 125: a North Thames Ovary Group Study. *Ann Oncol* **7**(4), 361–4.

Rustin G J, Nelstrop A E, Bentzen S M, Piccart M J *et al.* (1999). Use of tumour markers in monitoring the course of ovarian cancer. *Annals of Oncology* **10**(Suppl.1), 21–7.

Sandercock J, Parmar M K *et al.* (1998). First-line chemotherapy for advanced ovarian cancer: paclitaxel, cisplatin and the evidence. (See comments). *Br J Cancer* **78**(11), 1471–8.

Scoutt L M & McCarthy S M (1991). Imaging of ovarian masses: magnetic resonance imaging. *Clin Obstet Gynecol* **34**(2), 443–51.

Semelka R C, Lawrence P H *et al.* (1993). Primary ovarian cancer: prospective comparison of contrast-enhanced CT and pre and postcontrast, fat-suppressed MR imaging, with histologic correlation. *J Magn Reson Imaging* **3**(1), 99–106.

Stuart G, Bertelsen K *et al.* (1998). Updated analysis shows a highly significant improved overall survival (OS) for cisplatin-Paclitaxel as first line treatment of advanced ovarian cancer: mature results of the EORTC-GCCG, NOCOVA, NCIC, CTG and Scottish Intergroup Trial. *Proc ASCO* **17**, 361a.

Tuxen M K *et al.* (1995). Tumor markers in the management of patients with ovarian cancer. *Cancer Treatment Reviews* **21**, 215–45.

van der Burg M E, van Lent M *et al.* (1995). The effect of debulking surgery after induction chemotherapy on the prognosis in advanced epithelial ovarian cancer. Gynecological Cancer Cooperative Group of the European Organization for Research and Treatment of Cancer. (See comments). *N Engl J Med* **332**(10), 629–34.

Vermorken J B (1994). Consolidation therapy in patients with advanced ovarian cancer. *Eur J Gynaecol Oncol* **15**(1), 7–13.

Warwick J, Kehoe S *et al.* (1995). Long term follow-up of patients with ovarian cancer involved in clinical trials – important prognostic features. *British Journal of Cancer* **72**(6), 1513–17.

Chapter 6

The developing role of the oncology nurse specialist

Karen Maughan

Introduction

Clinical nurse specialists have traditionally had a strong role in the specialties of oncology and palliative care, and many of these posts have been 'pump-primed' by the UK charity, Macmillan Cancer Relief. This chapter aims to set the role of the oncology nurse specialist within the context of the nursing profession, and attempts to clarify the unique contribution of specialist nurses who are working with cancer patients.

Historically, the nursing profession has been hierarchically organised, rigidly segmented and preoccupied with titles and qualifications. The revolution in NHS management of the past decade has largely broken down these old hierarchies, and the movement of nurse training into higher educational institutions has created different challenges for the profession. One constant issue, however, is the multiplicity of nursing role descriptions. Indeed, with local diversity and the wide range of practice developments, the problem is getting worse (Bagnall 1996).

The general public, employers and the nursing profession itself, are understandably confused by the deluge of nursing titles and diversification of roles. It is now time to seek to change the traditional old-fashioned view of the nurse's role and to inform people about the way cancer care is increasingly being delivered.

Background to the oncology nurse specialist's role

Since the 1970s there has been increased awareness of the issues cancer patients face and what can be done to help. An example of this was the identification of unmet needs for psychological and practical support for women with breast cancer (Morris *et al.* 1977; MaGuire 1996). Some of the first UK clinical nurse specialists in breast and cancer care were employed in the hope that they might help to alleviate some of these problems.

The Macmillan Clinical Nurse Specialist Model was introduced in 1975 and has become a recognised model in the specialty of cancer and palliative care. This model has evolved and developed in response to changing health needs and professional developments (Webber 1997). The charity's aim is to equip a small workforce of specialist nurses, who have been educated and prepared with the relevant knowledge, expertise and skills, to provide specialist nursing care to cancer patients presenting with complex problems and needs. This presents the current problem for nursing. A 'specialist' is by title someone who is recognised as being an expert. Much as beauty is perceived in the eye of the beholder, so too is expertise. While choosing an expert is an entirely subjective process, it is likely to reflect the norms and values held within an organisation (Conway 1998). An example of this may be in gynaecological oncology, and the different values placed on clinical experience within a specialist nursing job description. The balance between general gynaecology and cancer experience differs between the cancer centres. So, who or what is an expert nurse? Would we know one if we saw one?

The United Kingdom Central Council for Nursing Midwifery and Health Visiting (UKCC) has been working for a number of years now to clarify what has been described as a 'post-registration qualification structure nightmare' (Castledine 1998). In order for a clear differentiation to be made between nurses practising within a specialty and those who are 'specialists', the UKCC emphasis is now on the *level of practice* and not the *type of role*.

Three levels of nursing practice had previously been outlined in *The future of professional practice* (UKCC 1994): *generalist; specialist;* and *advanced*. These were later replaced with two new levels of nursing practice. The first level is the present generalist domain, and the second is referred to as 'higher level' practice. Those practising at this higher level will include clinical nurse specialists in oncology and palliative care.

What is important to cancer care, the nursing profession, and the general public, is that a clear and robust framework is developed that will identify those nurses who are working at a higher level of clinical nursing competency. Indeed, there is strong support that this level of practice should be regulated and linked to the re-registration cycle currently in operation for all qualified nurses (Waller 1998). A steering group of UKCC members and external experts are currently taking forward a work programme (UKCC 1998) which aims to articulate this 'higher level' of practice, provide clear leadership on the issue and develop assessment and accreditation of this level through clinical practice and educational preparation.

Providing a structure for cancer nursing services

The Calman/Hine report (Department of Health 1995) has provided a strategic framework to help commissioners and providers of cancer services to make well informed and wise decisions. The creation of a network of care, from primary care, cancer units and cancer centres, would facilitate the organisation and delivery of a new, and better structure for the provision of cancer services. The report recommended that all cancer nursing services should be structured to ensure access to specialist nurses with:

- site-specific expertise (e.g. breast care, gynaecological cancer)
- specialist skills (e.g. lymphoedema management, chemotherapy administration)
- palliative care, counselling and psychosocial support
- stoma care.

The report did not, however, clearly articulate the nursing implications from the framework, but made a very broad statement recommending that patients should have access to nurses with appropriate experience and skills.

High-quality, integrated cancer services clearly depend upon the calibre of the health care professionals who deliver them and the collaborative way in which they work. A report on the workforce planning implications for cancer nursing (Royal College of Nursing 1996) recommended that strategic issues – for example, the development of good practice guidelines and the provision of good quality cancer and palliative care education – are paramount.

Guidelines devised by the Cancer Nursing Society of the Royal College of Nursing (Ferguson 1996) have explicitly stated that nurses caring for cancer patients in a cancer centre or unit should have a post-registration qualification in cancer care, and nurse specialists should be educated to degree or higher degree level. These, however, are neither realistic nor achievable at present, given that the Calman/Hine report failed to deal with issues of implementation, such as resources to provide adequately trained cancer nurses for the future. A report from the Cancer Collaboration (1996) has attempted an estimate of the required number of specialist nurses in cancer centres and units, although the report acknowledges that there are very few data on which to base these figures. It would appear that the NHS has, yet again, been asked to improve the quality and range of services without adequate information and financial support.

Corner (1996) states that nursing is ill prepared academically to meet the future challenges of cancer care, as fewer than 1 per cent of registered nurses in the UK have had any formal post-registration cancer training. According to a study by Ankrett (1997), which aimed to explore the current clinical nurse specialist resource within cancer centres, the current provision of specialist cancer nursing care is inequitable: while all oncology and palliative care nurse specialists in the study appeared to have the clinical experience needed to underpin their level of practice, deficits were found with regard to educational preparation for their role. Only 20 per cent of the sample fulfilled the requirements for specialist practice by holding degree level education, as recommended by the UKCC (1998). This has implications for current recruitment policies and educational pathways for existing oncology nurse specialists.

Education and training are a priority for cancer centres, as they have a responsibility to provide advanced cancer nursing education for those within and outside the centre. Information and co-ordination between the cancer centre and units are essential to ensure that all nursing staff have access to the same programmes of education. Accredited courses and in-house education should also be in alignment to prevent unnecessary duplication and safeguard standards. A key challenge for cancer nursing leaders is how to take forward a strategy that will address the current educational deficits, and will improve cancer nursing in the future by providing adequately prepared nursing personnel.

The oncology nurse specialist

The principles upon which oncology nurse specialists carry out their role lie in the fact that they are not primary carers: key to their role is to prepare primary carers (e.g. district nurses and ward staff) with the required skills and knowledge so that the highest standards of care can be made available to the greatest number of patients. The focus of this role is on clinical cancer expertise, education, research and management contribution to the multidisciplinary activities in either a hospital or community setting.

Macmillan Cancer Relief (Webber 1996) advises that nurse specialists should influence patient care by offering two kinds of service: direct and indirect care. These are examined below.

Direct care

Direct care is provided by the clinical nurse specialist at three levels:

• *Level 1* – includes assessment and planning for patients and their families at initial presentation. All registered nurses should be able to provide this level of care, and the nurse specialist intervention may focus on supporting staff to develop this basic level of competency.

• *Level 2* – competencies are required to work with patients and their families with regard to physical symptoms or psychological distress, which can be managed by implementing established interventions and protocols.

• *Level 3* – requires expertise to work with patients who have intractable and multifaceted needs and problems.

The aim of specialist nursing in gynaecological oncology, for example, is to promote optimal physical recovery following surgery and treatment. The reduction of anxiety, depression and sexual dysfunction through the provision of advice and counselling is often possible. Nursing intervention must be responsive to the individual needs of the woman and her partner, reflecting the different needs which arise at different points along the care continuum. The nurse needs to be proactive in discussing difficult issues with women – for example, sexual health concerns are often a difficult topic for women to discuss in the medical consultation.

The cancer patient travels on a journey from diagnosis towards cure or death. What is often encountered on this journey, for the patient, is a great deal of uncertainty about the future. There are often crisis points along the care continuum which may require the involvement of a nurse specialist. These are:

- distress at the time of diagnosis
- physiological and psychological effects of cancer, surgery and treatment
- changes in lifestyle and activities due to illness
- effect on family and friends
- other life issues (e.g. single parenthood, bereavement, financial hardship, divorce)
- recurrence of illness and more advancing disease
- pain and symptoms.

Cancer nurses accept that the expression of emotions and the disclosure of feelings may affect the cancer patient's ability to adjust to their diagnosis and cope with their treatment. They acknowledge, too, the potential power of communication to lessen the fear that often accompanies the 'cancer journey' (Richardson & Wilson-Barnett 1995). The quality of the nurse–patient relationship in cancer care is therefore important, as it is perhaps potentially the most therapeutic for the patient and their family.

Indirect care

The provision of training and education constitutes much of the indirect care provided by oncology nurse specialists. They may run in-house cancer education programmes, as well as contributing to diploma and degree level oncology and palliative care courses.

Most oncology nurse specialist job descriptions have a research remit, but while the educational component has blossomed, their research output remains a very low priority. This is possibly due to the fact they are already practising multiple roles. A study by Robichaud & Hamric (1986) indicates that the average time a nurse specialist devotes to research or audit activity is 2.2 per cent of the working week. It could be suggested that the ideal time a nurse specialist should spend engaged in research activity is approximately 15 per cent.

The fundamental task of cancer nursing research is the generation of a relevant knowledge base for cancer nursing practice, education and management, the primary focus of research being the impact of cancer and its treatment on the lives of patients and their families. Cancer nursing research is, therefore, clearly distinguishable from research undertaken by nurses who are acting as data collectors in medical research trials.

The need for a well-trained workforce to carry out research should be stressed. There is considerable support for the argument that the research base in nursing is so poorly developed, and the opportunities for funding so limited, that nursing should be regarded as a special case for resourcing and cultivating. This may present an opportunity. Clinical effectiveness as an initiative is explicitly intended to be a multidisciplinary, collaborative exercise. It could be argued that nursing research may flourish most readily in the multidisciplinary environment of health services research. What oncology nurse specialists need is access to national networks and contacts with other active researchers in clinical practice.

Oncology nurse specialists are ideally placed to facilitate a co-ordinated approach to research implementation, bringing together research evidence, clinical guidelines, clinical audit and outcome assessment. More importantly, integration of research findings into nursing practice is as much an issue of dissemination and persuasion as of method. The success of balancing direct and indirect components of the nurse specialist's role will be measurable in the developments within clinical practice.

Several components of the oncology nurse specialist's role have been described. Teaching, consultancy, leadership and research, however, are all functions that depend upon clinical expertise.

Conclusions

Clinical nurse specialists in cancer care are faced with both challenges and opportunities in the future. Nursing cannot move forward alone. Cancer services thrive with multidisciplinary and multi-agency collaboration and partnership. All health professionals, therefore, should have a vested interest in specialist nursing developments.

The oncology nurse specialist must be fully integrated, and an equal partner, in the system of health care delivery. Although direct care with patients is at the centre of this role, this should not be to the detriment of other indirect role components. The ability to influence cancer services at a strategic level should be acknowledged, as the specialist nurse can contribute to the development of cancer services within an organisation.

There is an opportunity for oncology nurse specialists to develop professionally towards being more recovery-oriented, with an emphasis on rehabilitation and adaptation. This implies a broader definition of health which is patient-centred and acknowledges the cancer patient fears for the future. For example, the giving of 'hope' would appear to be very important to patients and their family during the recovery period.

This is the 'new' nursing which can be characterised by: an emphasis on the patient as a person, thus acknowledging the psychological and social contexts of illness; an emphasis on health rather than cured illness, with the establishment of a therapeutic health care relationship as a constituent of the nursing role; and an emphasis on the nurse's role as patient advocate (Reed & Ground 1995).

For the oncology nurse specialist to function effectively, the ability to move across traditional boundaries is essential. For example, outpatients' clinics are not always conducive for providing information and counselling, and patients' stay in hospital is often too short to provide adequate psychological and social support. It could be argued, therefore, that nurse specialists must provide care at the point of need, regardless of whether the patient is at home or in hospital.

There are concerns, particularly by some community nursing staff, that they are being deskilled by specialist nurses. Raising the profile of the role of the specialist nurse in oncology and palliative care can do much to reassure staff that the service is complementary to the existing community services. Through the development of good working relationships, the nurse specialist may be seen as less of a threat, and more of a valuable resource to have available.

An integrated service, crossing the boundaries between primary and secondary care, is a wonderful opportunity for better communication and liaison. The oncology nurse specialist can potentially provide the 'stitching' to facilitate seamless cancer care.

Opportunities for experienced oncology and palliative care nurse specialists are currently limited, as there is no clear clinical career pathway available. Clinical expertise is subsequently lost to the NHS as nurse specialists develop their careers in general management or academia. Although the Government's intentions to develop clinical nurse consultant posts (NHS Executive 1998) should be greeted with caution, this new role may provide an alternative career path for experienced oncology nurse specialists who wish to advance their careers, but wish to retain day-to-day contact with patients.

References

Ankrett H (1997). *Exploration of the clinical nurse specialist resource in designated cancer centres in a health region and examination of the implications for the implementation of the Calman/Hine (1995) recommendations.* NHS Executive, London.

Bagnall P (1996). *The continuous development of nursing practice: a position paper.* The Queen's Nursing Institute, London.

Cancer Collaboration (1996). *The new cancer policy: workforce and training implications.* King's Fund, London.

Castledine G (1998). From specialist practice role to level of practice. *British Journal of Nursing* **7**(11), 682.

Conway J (1998). Evolution of the species 'expert nurse'. An examination of the practical knowledge held by expert nurses. *Journal of Clinical Nursing* **7**, 75–82.

Corner J (1996). Review: Cancer nursing services in Scotland – are we ready to meet the challenge? *Nursing Times Research* **1**(5), 381.

Department of Health (1995). *A policy framework for commissioning cancer services: a report of the expert advisory group on cancer to the Chief Medical Officers of England and Wales.* DoH, London.

Ferguson A (1996). *The workforce and planning implications for nursing and professionals allied to medicine of the Calman/Hine report – A policy framework for commissioning cancer services.* NHS Executive Northern and Yorkshire, Leeds.

MaGuire P G (1976). The psychological and social sequelae of mastectomy. In *Modern perspectives in the psychiatric aspects of surgery* (ed. J Howells). Churchill Livingstone, Edinburgh.

Morris T, Greer S & White P (1977). Psychological and social adjustment to mastectomy. *Cancer* **40**, 2381–7.

NHS Executive (1998). *Nurse consultants.* HSC 1998/161.

Reed J & Ground I (1995). *Philosophy for nursing*, p.151. Arnold, London.

Richardson A & Wilson-Barnett J (1995). Emotional disclosure between cancer patients and nurses. In *Nursing research in cancer care*, p.167. Scutari Press, London.

Robichaud A & Hamric A B (1986). Time documentation of clinical nurse specialist activities. *J Nurs Adm* **16**(1), 31–6.

Royal College of Nursing (1996). *A structure for cancer nursing services.* RCN, London.

UKCC (1994). *The future of professional practice: Council's standards for education and practice following education.* UKCC, London.

UKCC (1998). *A higher level of practice – consultation document.* UKCC, London.

Waller S (1998). Clarifying the UKCC's position in relation to higher level practice. *British Journal of Nursing* **7**(16), 960.

Webber J (1996). *The evolving role of the Macmillan nurse.* Cancer Relief Macmillan Fund, London.

Webber J (1997). *Macmillan clinical nurse specialist – position statement.* Macmillan Cancer Relief, London.

Chapter 7

Surgery in ovarian cancer: defining the rules

David Luesley

Introduction

The objectives of surgical intervention in ovarian cancer are quite clear and simple: to achieve an accurate diagnosis and assessment of disease extent and to eradicate or palliate disease either by surgical intervention alone or as part of a planned multidisciplinary approach. These objectives should, ideally, be achieved with minimal morbidity to the patient and without adversely affecting physical and/or psychological outcomes.

Achieving such objectives is less simple than formulating them. The 'rules', in effect, are the conventions within which surgical interventions are planned and conducted. These conventions are based upon experience, consensus and evidence, and as will be demonstrated, many lack robust data to support them.

The roles of surgery

The roles of surgery vary: they range from a simple diagnostic laparoscopy to an extensive laparotomy that may entail bowel and splenic resection. If ovarian cancer is suspected, and the majority of cases can be by a combination of clinical examination, imaging and use of tumour markers, then cases should be managed by teams with the appropriate training and expertise.

Diagnosis and assessment of disease

Traditionally, diagnosis and assessment have been by a formal staging laparotomy at which time a tissue diagnosis was achieved, the stage assessed and then formal excision of disease undertaken. It is not surprising that with several roles combined there is scope for variations within the predefined conventions. Current consensus still dictates that a laparotomy through a mid-line incision should be performed. This allows access to the upper abdomen and a thorough tactile and visual inspection of all of the peritoneal surfaces. Suspicious areas should be subjected to biopsy and, if no ascites is present, then lavage with warmed normal saline should be performed. As the current staging system (FIGO) includes the status of the retroperitoneal lymph nodes, then these should also be biopsied.

There are several studies already published indicating that a rigorous approach to staging results in an upstaging phenomenon but as yet no relationship between the adequacy of staging and survival. Indeed one author, focusing on stage I disease, was unable to demonstrate any difference in survival between groups adjudged to have been staged adequately and those who were not (Finn *et al.* 1992). This study, although retrospective, was a registry-based review, and thus avoided referral bias. Nevertheless, the outcome should be assessed with care. Adequate staging should, however, be supported on grounds of good clinical practice as it is unlikely to prejudice the care of patients and may yet be shown to be of benefit.

Diagnosis depends upon histopathology. The use of frozen sections remains somewhat controversial and thus during surgery decisions may have to be based upon the suspected nature of disease. There are occasions when it may be impossible to determine whether the condition is malignant or not and indeed the organ of origin. Where sufficient doubt exists, the surgeon should do the minimum to make a diagnosis and provide immediate palliation. While this might necessitate further surgical intervention in the event of malignancy being confirmed by histopathology, it avoids the tragedy of pelvic clearances in women with endometriosis or germ cell tumours who might wish to retain fertility; it also avoids unnecessary extensive surgery in women who may have disseminated intraperitoneal malignancy from gastrointestinal malignancies. Intra-operative decision making is an important aspect of surgical management in this condition and naturally should be included in pre-operative counselling. Most, if not all, women will fully understand the need for a subsequent laparotomy if the reasoning is fully explained to them prior to initial surgery.

Removing disease

When future fertility is not an issue and where there are reasonable grounds to suspect malignancy, the current consensus is to perform a total hysterectomy and bilateral salpingo-oophorectomy. In addition, as part of staging, any other suspicious lesions should be biopsied – retroperitoneal nodal biopsies, peritoneal lavage and at least an infracolic omentectomy. Total macroscopic clearance of disease is the ultimate goal but it is a goal that is not always attainable.

There are several possible scenarios. First, in women who have either completed childbearing or when future fertility is no longer an issue:

• The abdomen is normal apart from an enlarged but otherwise normal ovary. In this situation the likelihood is either a benign ovarian cyst, a borderline tumour or stage I disease. The objectives of appropriate diagnosis and staging can be achieved by TAH and BSO, with relevant biopsies, washings, etc. In exceptional circumstances, removal of the affected appendage may suffice, although there remains the risk of occult disease in the remaining ovary.

• There is an obvious malignant tumour arising from one or both appendages but no evidence of further abdominal involvement. Again, the objective laid down by convention may be met by total abdominal hysterectomy (TAH) and bilateral salpingo-oophorectomy (BSO) with relevant biopsies, washings, etc.

• There is an obvious ovarian primary with peritoneal spread of disease. There is now sufficient evidence to suggest that women who have no macroscopic disease following surgery fare better than those who have (Ozols 1991; Potter *et al.* 1991; Hoskins *et al.* 1992; Hacker & van der Berg 1993). This is the basis for cytoreduction (see below). If all tumour can be removed, then this should be attempted. The dilemma arises when this is not considered possible.

• There is intra-abdominal carcinomatosis and the ovary is not the obvious source of the primary. There are no data to suggest that attempting TAH and BSO with macroscopic clearance will be of benefit in this situation. Both removal of the ovaries and representative biopsies are advised in this situation more from a diagnostic than a therapeutic perspective.

The next group of scenarios applies to women who would wish, if possible, to retain their reproductive capacity. These women will usually be younger and will contain non-epithelial and borderline tumours where there may be alternative methods of disease management or where radical cytoreductive surgery is unnecessary. It is in this group that there is a greater likelihood of doing less at the primary laparotomy and a consequent increase in the risk of requiring a further laparotomy. Part of the pre-operative assessment should include serum markers, not just CA 125, but also ßHCG and alphafetoprotein. Even with the use of these markers, many non-epithelial tumours will have normal levels so reliance on negative markers should be avoided.

In these patients the primary surgery should aim to provide a diagnosis, gauge extent of disease, provide the basis for palliation of the presenting symptoms but aim to conserve at least one ovary, the uterus and tube. There is no advantage of total pelvic clearance over unilateral salpingo-oophorectomy in terms of survival (Gershenson 1992). There is ample evidence to suggest that non-surgical approaches to the management of germ cell tumours result in good outcomes in terms of survival and conserve fertility (Williams *et al.* 1998). The same is true to a certain extent with lymphomas affecting the ovary. The long-term risk in women who have fertility-sparing surgery with unilateral borderline tumours is less certain

(Trimble & Trimble 1993; Barnhill *et al.* 1995). Whether the remaining ovary should be removed after completion of childbearing is a valid question and the answer must consider not only perceived risk but the patient's anxieties and perceptions. Where fertility-sparing surgery has been performed and the eventual diagnosis is confirmed as epithelial, then the decision is whether to remove the remaining pelvic organs or to follow conservatively. There are insufficient data to be dogmatic with regard to stage Ia disease; the current consensus, however, would be to err on the side of caution and offer total pelvic clearance in all but some stage Ia tumours.

Primary debulking

Of all the interventions in epithelial ovarian cancer, the role of primary cytoreduction remains the most contentious. Is the volume of residual disease achievable after surgery a function of surgical effort or permissive tumour biology? In other words, is any recordable survival benefit inherent in the tumour rather than a result of cytoreduction itself? Removing tumour to achieve a maximum diameter of less than 2 cm is achievable in 23–77 per cent of cases using conventional surgical techniques (Chen & Bochner 1985; Piver & Baker 1986; Unzelman 1992; Nelson *et al.* 1993; Rodriguez *et al.* 1994), and after secondary procedures this figure improves to 39–77 per cent (Jacob *et al.* 1991; Goodman *et al.* 1992; Segna *et al.* 1993). Employing ultraradical dissection techniques these figures can be increased to 95.7–100 per cent (Deppe *et al.* 1989; Adelson 1992; Eisenkop *et al.* 1993; Guidozzi & Ball 1994; Fanning & Hilgers 1995; Scarabelli *et al.* 1995). High, and some might say unacceptable, morbidity has been associated with these procedures (19.1–42 per cent) with an operative mortality of 2–3 per cent (Piver & Baker 1986). To date no prospective randomised trials have been completed which demonstrate conclusively an improvement in survival from radical debulking and the debate concerning the clinical utility of cytoreduction will continue until robust evidence becomes available. The logistic difficulties that gynaecological oncologists have encountered in order to try to acquire such data suggest that the debate will be prolonged.

Advocates of primary partial cytoreduction, while citing observational data, admit that the relationship between surgical effort and survival is tenuous at best, but that there may be other important but theoretical reasons for considering debulking. One is based on the Goldie-Coldman hypothesis and the theoretical grounds that decreased tumour bulk leads to improved efficiency of chemotherapeutic regimens by removing areas of poor vascularity/oxygenation and consequently increasing the fraction of cycling/chemosensitive cells (Goldie & Coldman 1979; Skipper 1983). The converse should also be considered possible, i.e. that surgery may adversely affect the host tumour interface (Kehoe *et al.* 1995).

Cytoreduction trials

Accurate measurement of residual tumour volume and the standardisation of surgery, adjuvant therapy and biological tumour variables pose major problems in trial design. Several studies have been reported where response rates to chemotherapy and survival following optimal cytoreduction to below 0.5, 1.0, 1.5 or 2.0 cm are quoted (Griffiths 1975; Wharton & Herson 1981; Hacker et al. 1983; Heinz et al. 1988; Eisenkop et al. 1993) but reliable comparisons between these studies are difficult to draw when the aim of optimal cytoreduction varies by as much as 400 per cent. Small peritoneal seedlings which may often extend into hidden or poorly accessible areas plainly make residual tumour measurement inaccurate and should be questioned. In one interesting and underquoted study (Préfontaine et al. 1994), it was possible to demonstrate wide variations in the accuracy of measuring intraperitoneal nodules in a model system. Medical students and experienced gynaecologists found similar degrees of difficulty and wide variation in the assessment of 'nodules' in this model system.

Current imaging technologies have limitations in terms of resolution and the measurement of CA 125 or other tumour markers clearly gives no information related to individual seedling size. As such importance has been attached to the size of each residual seedling, agreement needs to be reached on standardisation of techniques of measurement and of optimal seedling size. In the author's opinion, total macroscopic clearance should be regarded as the only gold standard. This endpoint is at least reproducible even if not achievable in many cases. A case-control study containing small numbers (Eisenkop et al. 1993) has demonstrated a small but statistical survival advantage of total macroscopic clearance over optimal cytoreduction to below or equal to 1 cm – the authors themselves, however, calling for a randomised prospective trial to confirm their results. The Netherlands Joint Ovarian Cancer Study Group has reported a similar experience. Patients with a complete response at second-look laparotomy experienced a longer disease/therapy-free interval compared with patients achieving only a partial response or with microscopic disease at second-look laparotomy.

Most of the earlier studies of primary cytoreduction employed either single-agent or combination chemotherapy with alkylating agents and melphalan, but did not include platinum agents. It has been suggested that the type of chemotherapy and intrinsic tumour chemosensitivity may be equally or more important than cytoreduction in influencing median survival. Jacobs et al. (1988) certainly found in their small series that residual disease status was a prognostic variable but in a univariate analysis, dose intensity for cisplatin and doxorubicin also had prognostic value. Hunter et al. (1992), reviewing 58 studies, performed a multiple linear regression analysis on 6,962 patients. The result of this analysis showed that the survival effect of platinum-based chemotherapy was not related to the degree of maximum cytoreductive surgery. Other published data seem to support the concept of inherent chemosensitivity being more important than surgical resectability. The first comes from a study of neoadjuvant chemotherapy (Surwit *et al.* 1996). This was a retrospective review of 29 women selected over a six-year period. All had bulky advanced disease and were treated with either cisplatin or carboplatin prior to definitive surgery. Computed tomography, conventional radiography and clinical examination were the criteria upon which unlikely optimal primary resection was based. All but one patient had ascites and eight had stage IV disease by virtue of having a pleural effusion. A maximum of three courses of platinum were given and surgery took place within four weeks of the final course. The response was documented by clinical and tumour marker strategies (CA 125). There was a 2 log fall in the CA 125 in 11 patients (38 per cent) and all were optimally debulked to less than 1 cm residual disease. In seven patients (24 per cent) there was a 1 log fall in CA 125, and five of these were optimally debulked. None of the remaining patients achieved an optimally debulked status and their median survival was 18 months compared to 37 months in those achieving a greater than 2 log fall in CA 125. Overall 16 (55 per cent) women were optimally debulked after neoadjuvant chemotherapy, four undergoing bowel resection. Those undergoing bowel resection to achieve optimal cytoreduction had a similar survival to those who were only biopsied. The authors conclude that this schedule offers similar outcomes to women having adjuvant chemotherapy with interval debulking yet with only one operative procedure. Although not stated, it would also appear that tumour chemosensitivity would appear to be of major importance given the strong association between falling marker and survival. It would have been of value to know how much residual disease these good responders had following neoadjuvant treatment and whether or not surgery provided any additional benefit. This retrospective report provides yet more evidence in support of chemosensitivity, not surgical debulking, as being of primary importance in the outcome for women with advanced epithelial ovarian cancer.

A second small study reported by Kehoe *et al.* (1996) examined the outcome in women who had minimal primary surgery. They were selected usually on grounds of maximal debulking requiring at least two bowel and/or major organ resections; and even if this were possible they would still have had widespread residual disease with a maximum diameter greater than 2 cm. The overall median survival in this group of 29 patients was 17 months, but 29 months in those who demonstrated a response to platinum-containing chemotherapy. Studies such as these, with their conclusions strongly supportive of the chemosensitivity argument, are already prompting a resurgence of interest in properly designed neoadjuvant studies.

A further role for partial or optimal cytoreduction is that it provides a rapid means of palliation. This is an important issue given the increased priority accorded to palliative strategies in a disease situation with poor short-to-medium-term outcome. Furthermore, few, if any, reported trials have attempted to measure palliative effect (largely because of difficulties in measuring palliation). One study has, however, shown that patients undergoing a radical attempt at debulking appeared to enjoy benefit in terms of total days in hospital and return to normal daily activities (Blythe & Wahl 1982). This, however, was a relatively small uncontrolled study, although its importance lies in its attempt to bring palliative issues to the fore.

Secondary debulking

No other intra-abdominal malignancy has been associated with multiple laparotomies as much as epithelial ovarian cancer. Several factors have contributed to this. The first and perhaps most obvious is the relative infrequency with which even advanced ovarian cancer spreads outside the peritoneum. The second is the persisting belief in surgical reduction of tumour volume as being crucial to chemoresponse. A third consideration is the perceived need to offer surgical palliation when all else fails. Finally, there is a wealth of observational data demonstrating that the majority of patients presenting with advanced epithelial ovarian cancer will have intra-abdominal disease not only during but at the completion of primary chemotherapy.

If one collates data from published series on second-look laparotomy, over three-quarters of these patients will have evidence of macroscopic disease (Lippman et al. 1988; Luesley et al. 1988; Podratz et al. 1988; Hoskins et al. 1989; Lawton et al. 1990; Chamber et al. 1998). This would imply that secondary cytoreduction might have some utility in further reducing tumour mass. The caveat here, however, is that second-look procedures have been performed for a variety of indications; thus this group must be, by definition, very heterogeneous. Using similar collated data but only in platinum-exposed patients, only 29 per cent of patients were left with 'suboptimal' residual disease following attempted debulking either after or during chemotherapy (Lippman et al. 1988; Luesley et al. 1988; Podratz et al. 1988; Hoskins et al. 1989; Lawton et al. 1990; Chamber et al. 1998). While these data suggest that disease is present both during and after completion of chemotherapy in the majority of advanced epithelial ovarian cancer patients and that surgery is feasible and can resect, to an extent, to render the majority 'optimal', the data do not directly suggest that such intervention is advantageous in terms of survival. One could still be assessing a disease or chemotherapy effect, thus randomised trials are required.

Several authors have suggested that debulking at second-look laparotomy is advantageous in terms of survival in that survival is related to the volume of residual disease:

- Phillips et al. (1979) re-explored 65 patients after completing chemotherapy.

Fourteen were aggressively debulked and had a median survival of 31 months. All, however, were chemoresponders.

• Schwartz & Smith (1980) reported on a series of epithelial ovarian cancer patients having second-look procedures but the indications for the procedure were inconsistent. Initially it was performed in a 'neoadjuvant' setting, but the later patients were those experiencing toxicity on chemotherapy. Although platinum-based chemotherapy was not used in this study, there was little difference in outcome between total and partial resections. Patients progressing on chemotherapy appeared to do worse than those responding.

• Berek *at al.* (1983) had a mixed patient population: some had 'true' second-look operations (clinically in remission after chemotherapy), some were re-explored because of symptomatic obstruction, and some had planned cytoreduction because of persistent palpable tumour. As the total group numbered only 32, analysis by subgroups was not realistic. The authors, however, did recognise the importance of multiple variables other than post-resection volume.

• Bertelsen (1990) studied 361 patients with stage III and IV disease. Two hundred and seventeen had a second-look procedure and 94 of these had macroscopic tumour prior to surgery. Thirty-five patients were optimally debulked and 80 per cent of these were classified as chemoresponders; the response status of the remaining 59 was not immediately apparent but at least 36 per cent demonstrated progression. It is doubtful therefore that the groups were similar.

Not all uncontrolled data that have been published support the concept of secondary volume reduction being implicated in enhanced survival. Raju's study included 65 patients (Raju *et al.* 1982). Partial responders to chemotherapy who were converted to complete responders by the addition of cytoreduction at second laparotomy had a similar survival to those who were not totally debulked. Luesley *et al.* (1988) in their randomised trial of second-look versus no second-look after single-agent cisplatin could not show any survival advantage in the surgical arm. This study, however, was not specifically designed to assess the clinical utility of intervention debulking, which in this context is defined as a planned laparotomy performed during primary chemotherapy in patients adjudged to be responding to that chemotherapy.

There have been two published prospective randomised controlled trials assessing the survival advantage of intervention debulking and thus we are somewhat more fortunate than in the primary debulking scenario. The first by Redman *et al.* (1994) was designed to determine whether secondary cytoreduction performed during the course of the chemotherapy might improve survival. The hypothesis that the risk of chemoresistance developing spontaneously in tumour cells is a function of time was the rationale upon which this trial was based. Seventy-nine patients were prospectively randomised to receive either early cytoreduction (intervention debulking surgery (IDS)) after three courses of cisplatinum-based chemotherapy or no IDS. Only patients in whom the operating surgeon at the primary laparotomy felt that there was scope for further cytoreduction and in whom there was an objective response to chemotherapy were subjected to intervention. This was in retrospect a design error, as randomisation took place at the outset and thus many patients who did not fulfil the response criteria were excluded from IDS. Although the intention-to-treat design was appropriate, the power calculations did not fully take account of the likely number of women who would not eventually receive their randomised treatment option. The median survival in the IDS group was 15 months and in the non-IDS group 12 months, the difference being non-significant.

The second larger study was published in 1995 (van der Burg *et al.* 1995). This large prospective randomised trial has been recognised as a major contribution to the literature on this subject and was performed as a multicentre study under the auspices of the EORTC Gynaecological Cancer Co-operative Group. Surgical trials are difficult to plan, recruit to and monitor and all have their imperfections. This trial is no exception. Over a six-year period 425 women with advanced ovarian cancer who had suboptimal residual disease were enrolled into this study. Randomisation, however, took place after the completion of induction chemotherapy (platinum and cyclophosphamide). Only 319 patients underwent randomisation and only 278 had follow-up data complete at the time of reporting. Eventually, 130 patients had interval debulking and 138 did not. Eight-four per cent in each group completed the schedule of treatment (chemotherapy). No excess treatment-related morbidity was associated with interval debulking. Surgical data were missing on three patients and, of the 127 with data, 83 (65 per cent) had tumours greater than 1 cm (i.e. might possibly benefit from further tumour removal). Thirty-seven of these 83 patients (45 per cent) underwent cytoreduction to less than 1 cm. At the conclusion of treatment (induction chemotherapy followed by surgery or no surgery, then three more courses of chemotherapy), 70 per cent of the surgical group and 35 per cent of the non-surgical group had a complete response. The outcome measures all showed a significant positive advantage for those having debulking surgery, with a six-month advantage median survival and 56 versus 46 per cent alive at two years.

Although there may be a subgroup of patients who might benefit in terms of short-to-medium-term survival from further attempts at surgical cytoreduction, it by no means applies to all ovarian cancer patients. This trial had an accrual target of 440 randomised patients. This target was not achieved and, because of the known likely drop-out rates, should have been analysed on an intention-to-treat basis and the sample size inflated accordingly. Only 37 patients actually received the planned intervention (optimal cytoreduction), yet in those who underwent a failed attempt at cytoreduction, the results were similar to, if not worse than, the non-surgical group, raising the possibility of an adverse effect in certain patients. There is still a great deal to do before we can become more confident about the role of surgery in ovarian cancer. This trial, although far from perfect, is an important step towards achieving this goal.

Palliative surgery

Surgical intent may be classified as diagnostic, therapeutic and palliative. All therapeutic intent should palliate (i.e. have symptom control as at least one of its objectives), yet all palliative procedures are not therapeutic (i.e. disease eradication is not the primary goal). Some might argue that all surgery in epithelial ovarian cancer is palliative. This is probably an extreme view but, in advanced disease, the importance of the palliative aspect of a surgical procedure should not be underestimated. For the purposes of this chapter, palliative surgery is defined as a planned procedure whose primary intent is to alleviate a symptom or symptoms. A small group of patients might also be considered for what has become known as 'salvage' surgery. In this scenario, the objective is to remove large-volume 'localised' disease that may or may not be symptomatic where no alternative means of volume reduction is available (Wiltshaw *et al.* 1987).

Gastrointestinal obstruction

Gastrointestinal obstruction is a relatively frequent accompaniment to advanced incurable disease (Tunca *et al.* 1981; Beattie *et al.* 1989; Larson *et al.* 1989). Mechanical compression of the bowel and infiltration of the mesenteries alone or in combination and often at more than one site lead to progressive bowel dysfunction (Addison 1983; Ripamonti 1994). Usually, medical measures should be employed initially but, if symptoms fail to resolve and there is a reasonable expectation of survival more than two months, then surgery should be considered (Rubin *et al.* 1989). Before even considering surgical intervention several criteria should be considered. These include:

- surgery must achieve the symptomatic goal
- there must be low procedure-related morbidity
- there must be minimal interference with subsequent quality of life.

Several surgical options can be considered to try to meet these criteria and include: gastrostomy; jejunostomy; iliostomy (loop and terminal); colostomy (loop, transverse, descending and sigmoid); end-colostomy; entero-enterostomy; and resection and re-anastamosis.

Defining a 'useful outcome' has been difficult but most who have published on this subject agree that survival beyond 60 days should be considered useful palliation. Using this type of definition Krebs & Goplerud (1983) reported an operative mortality (death within 30 days) of 12 per cent and no benefit (deaths within 8 weeks) in 35 per cent. Redman *et al.* (1988) reported similar figures of 15 and 38 per cent respectively. These figures certainly support a role for this type of intervention but highlight the difficulties in case selection. It would appear that single-site and low-level obstruction cases fare better than those with multiple-level site obstruction. Other patient and disease characteristics would also seem important and, based upon these, Krebs *et al.* (1989) formulated a scoring system that could be applied pre-operatively in an attempt to select those cases where surgery might result in a more favourable outcome. Table 7.1 shows their scoring system.

Table 7.1 Scoring system

Variable	Category	Score
Age	<45 years	0
	45–65 years	1
	>65 years	2
Nutritional status	Minimally deprived	0
	Moderately deprived	1
	Severely deprived	2
Tumour status	No palpable abdominal masses	0
	Palpable abdominal masses	1
	Liver or distant metastases	2
Ascites	None or minimal	0
	Moderate	1
	Severe (symptomatic/frequent tap)	2
Previous chemotherapy	None (no adequate trial)	0
	Failed single-agent	1
	Failed combination	2
Previous radiation therapy	None	0
	Pelvic only	1
	Whole abdomen	2

[*Source:* Krebs *et al.* 1989]

By applying this scoring system to their patients, Krebs *et al.* were able to show a relationship between pre-operative score and subsequent survival (Figure 7.1).

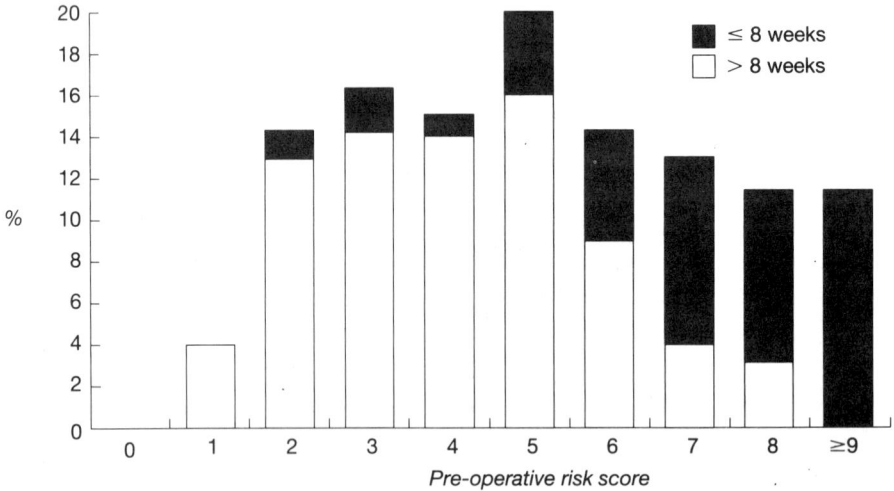

Figure 7.1 The relationship between 'pre-operative score' and survival following surgery

A score of six or less appears to offer the optimal cut-off point and, applying this to a separate series of patients, Gadducci *et al.* (1998) were able to confirm the clinical utility. In their series of 67 consecutive cases of epithelial ovarian cancer, 34 developed intestinal obstruction during the course of their disease. Nineteen had a score of 6 or less, the remainder greater than 6. The median interval between diagnosis to obstruction was 19.5 months. Among the surgically treated patients in this study, the median survival was 215 days for the 16 patients with an optimal score. Only eight patients with a suboptimal score actually received surgery and the overall median survival in the poor-score patients was 36 days. Ten of the 22 patients having further surgery received further chemotherapy, whereas 12 did not and the median survival in relation to post-operative treatment was 275 versus 45 days. This of course confuses the issue a little. Was it the further chemotherapy or the surgery that improved the palliative prospects? Certainly, if surgery led to sufficient improvement to allow meaningful further chemotherapy to be given, then it is probably of value.

It is unlikely that randomised trials will be performed to assess the palliative value of surgery, largely because of the priority to offer meaningful symptomatic relief.

Conclusions

Surgery still has a very major role to play in the management of women with epithelial ovarian cancer. Early disease can be satisfactorily managed by surgery with or without the use of subsequent chemotherapy, furthermore there is scope to offer fertility-sparing surgery in early disease, although no data as yet support ovarian conservation in unilateral stage I epithelial ovarian cancer or indeed borderline. There are, however, reported cases of ovarian conservation, particularly those with non-epithelial tumours.

Total macroscopic clearance at primary surgery should still remain as the ideal and surgeons should not discount the palliative aspects of the first laparotomy. Optimal cytoreduction still requires robust proof, more so perhaps in the primary setting than in the secondary setting, although here also confirmatory data are required before embarking on wide-scale intervention debulking surgery. This type of operation should remain, for the time being, within the realms of research protocols.

Exploratory or diagnostic laparotomy performed after the end of a course of chemotherapy should be discouraged, as it has no demonstrable utility in improving survival. Even within the confines of a clinical trial one might argue that it has little value.

Palliative surgery has a role and observational studies would appear to be moving towards refining such a role. It is unlikely that more solid data based upon randomisation will be available to guide clinicians in this area.

References

Addison N V (1983). Pseudo-obstruction of the large bowel. *Journal of the Royal Society of Medicine* **76**, 252–5.

Adelson M (1992). Ultrasonic surgical aspirator in cytoreduction of splenic metastases to avoid splenectomy. *Journal of Reproductive Medicine* **37**(11), 917–20.

Barnhill D R, Kurman R J, Brady M F et al. (1995). Preliminary analysis of the behaviour of stage I ovarian serous tumours of low malignant potential: a Gynecologic Oncology Group Study. *Journal of Clinical Oncology* **3**, 2752–5.

Beattie G J, Leonard R & Smith J F (1989). Bowel obstruction in ovarian carcinoma: a retrospective study and review of the literature. *Journal of Palliative Care* **3**, 275–80.

Berek J S, Hacker N F, Lagasse L D, Nieberg R K & Elashoff R M (1983). Survival of patients following secondary cytoreductive surgery in ovarian cancer. *Obstetrics and Gynecology* **61**(2), 189–93.

Bertelsen K (1990). Tumour reduction surgery and long term survival in advanced ovarian cancer; a DACOVA study. *Gynecologic Oncology* **38**, 203–9.

Blythe J G & Wahl T P (1982). Debulking surgery: does it improve the quality of survival? *Gynecologic Oncology* **14**, 396–408.

Chambers S, Chambers J T, Kohorn E I et al. (1988). Evaluation of the role of second look surgery in ovarian cancer. *Obstetrics and Gynecology* **72**, 404–9.

Chen S & Bochner R (1985). Assessment of morbidity and mortality in primary cytoreductive surgery for advanced ovarian carcinoma. *Gynecologic Oncology* **20**, 190–5.

Deppe G, Malviya V K, Boike G & Malone J M Jr (1989). Use of cavitron surgical aspirator for debulking of diaphragmatic metastases in patients with advanced ovarian carcinoma. Surgery, *Gynecology and Obstetrics* **168**, 455–8.

Eisenkop S M, Nalick R H, Wang H J & Teng N N (1993). Peritoneal implant elimination during cytoreductive surgery for ovarian cancer: impact on survival. *Gynecologic Oncology* 51(**2**), 224–9.

Fanning J & Hilgers R D (1995). Loop electrosurgical excision procedure for intensified cytoreduction of ovarian cancer. *Gynecologic Oncology* **57**, 188–92.

Finn C B, Luesley D M, Buxton E J et al. (1992). Is Stage I epithelial ovarian cancer overtreated both surgically and systemically ? Results of a five year cancer registry review. *British Journal of Obstetrics and Gynæcology* 99(**1**), 154–5.

Gadducci A, Iacconi P, Fanucchi A, Cosio S, Miccoli P & Genazzani A R (1998). Survival after intestinal obstruction in patients with fatal ovarian cancer: Analysis of prognostic variables. *International Journal of Gynecologic Cancer* 8(**3**), 177–82.

Gershenson D M (1992). Malignant germ cell tumours of the ovary: clinical features and management. In *Gynecologic oncology*, 2nd edn, vol.2 (ed. M Coppleson, Monaghan & Tattersall), pp.935–46. Churchill Livingstone, Edinburgh.

Goldie J & Coldman A (1979). A mathematical model for relating the drug sensitivity of tumour to their spontaneous mutation rate. *Cancer Treatment Reviews* **63**, 1727–9.

Goodman H, Harlow B, Sheets E et al. (1992). The role of cytoreductive surgery in the management of stage IV epithelial ovarian carcinoma. *Gynecologic Oncology* 46(**3**), 367–71.

Griffiths C (1975). *Surgical resection of tumour bulk in the primary treatment of ovarian carcinoma. Symposium on ovarian cancer.* National Cancer Institute Monographs **42**, 1010–14.

Guidozzi F & Ball J H (1994). Extensive primary cytoreductive surgery for advanced epithelial ovarian cancer. *Gynecologic Oncology* 53(**3**), 326–30.

Hacker N F & van der Berg M E (1993). Advanced ovarian cancer. Debulking and intervention surgery. *Annals of Oncology* **4** (Suppl.4), 17–22.

Hacker N, Berek J, Lagasse L, Nieberg R & Elashoff R (1983). Primary cytoreductive surgery for epithelial ovarian carcinoma. *Obstetrics and Gynecology* **61**, 413–20.

Heintz A, Van Oosterom A, Trimbos J, Schaberg A, Van de Velde E & Nooy M (1988). The treatment of advanced ovarian carcinoma (1). Clinical variables associated with prognosis. *Gynecologic Oncology* 30(**3**), 347–58.

Hoskins W J, Rubin S C, Dulaney E et al. (1989). Influence of secondary cytoreduction at the time of second look laparotomy on the survival of patients with epithelial ovarian cancer. *Gynecologic Oncology* **34**, 365–71.

Hoskins W J, Bundy B N, Thigpen J T & Omura G A (1992). The influence of cytoreductive surgery on recurrence free interval and survival in small volume stage III epithelial ovarian cancer: a Gynecologic Oncology Group study. *Gynecologic Oncology* 47(**2**), 159–66.

Hunter R W, Alexander N D & Soutter W P (1992). Meta-analysis of surgery in advanced ovarian carcinoma: is maximum cytoreductive surgery an independent determinant of prognosis? *American Journal of Obstetrics and Gynecology* 166(**2**), 504–11.

Jacobs A, Sommers G, Homan S et al. (1988). 31, 233–45. GO. Therapy of ovarian carcinoma: the relationship of dose level and treatment intensity to survival. *Gynecologic Oncology* **31**, 233–45.

Jacob J, Gershenson D, Morris M, Copeland L, Burke T & Wharton J (1991). Neoadjuvant chemotherapy and interval debulking for advanced epithelial ovarian cancer. *Gynecologic Oncology* 42(**2**), 146–50.

Kehoe S T, Luesley D M, Ward K & Chan K K (1995). In vivo evidence of increased malignant cell proliferation following surgery in ovarian cancer. *International Journal of Gynecologic Cancer* **5**, 121–8.

Kehoe S T, Herod J, Van Geene P et al. (1996). Intentional non-radical surgery and survival in advanced ovarian cancer: results of a pilot study. *International Journal of Gynecologic Cancer* 6(**6**), 448–51.

Krebs H B & Goplerud D R (1983). Surgical management of bowel obstruction in advanced ovarian carcinoma. *Obstetrics and Gynecology* **61**, 327–30.

Krebs H B & Helmkamp F (1989). Management of intestinal obstruction in ovarian cancer. *Oncology* **3**, 25–31.

Larson J E, Podczaski E S, Manetta A, Whitney C W & Mortel R (1989). Bowel obstruction in patients with ovarian carcinoma: analysis of prognostic factors. *Gynecologic Oncology* **35**, 61–5.

Lawton F, Luesley D, Redman C, Chan K K, Varma R & Blackledge G (1990). Feasibility and outcome of complete secondary tumor resection for patients with advanced ovarian cancer. *J Surg Oncol*

Lippman S M, Alberts D s & Slymen D J (1988). Second look laparotomy in epithelial ovarian cancer. *Cancer* **61**, 2571–6.

Luesley D M, Lawton F G, Blackledge G et al. (1988). Failure of second look laparotomy to influence survival in epithelial ovarian cancer. *Lancet* **2**, 599–603.

Nelson B, Rosenfield A & Schwartz P (1993). Preoperative abdominopelvic computed tomographic prediction of optimal cytoreduction in epithelial ovarian carcinoma. *Journal of Clinical Oncology* 11(**1**), 166–72.

Ozols R F (1991). Ovarian cancer: new clinical approaches. *Cancer Trea Rev* **18**, 77–83.

Phillips B P, Buschbaum H J & Lifshitz S (1979). Re-exploration after treatment for ovarian carcinoma. *Gynecologic Oncology* **8**, 339–45.

Piver M & Baker T (1986). The potential for optimal (≤2 cm) cytoreductive surgery in advanced ovarian carcinoma at a tertiary medical centre: a prospective study. *Gynecologic Oncology* **24**, 1–8.

Podratz K C, Schray M F, Wieand H S et al. (1988). Evaluation of treatment and survival after positive second look laparotomy. *Gynecologic Oncology* **31**, 9–24.

Potter M E, Partridge E E, Hatch K, Soong Seng-Saw, Austin J M, Shingleton HM (1991). Primary surgical therapy of ovarian cancer: how much and when. *Gynecologic Oncology* **40**, 195–200.

Préfontaine M, Gelfand A T, Donovan J T & Powell J L (1994). Reproducibility of tumour measurements in ovarian cancer: a study of interobserver variability. *Gynecologic Oncology* **55**, 87–90.

Raju K S, McKinna J A, Barker G H et al. (1982). Second look operations in the planned management of advanced ovarian cancer. *American Journal of Obstetrics and Gynecology* **144**, 650–4.

Redman C W E, Shafi M I, Lawton F G et al. (1988). Survival following intestinal obstruction in ovarian cancer. *European Journal of Surgical Oncology* **14**, 383–6.

Redman C, Warwick J, Luesley D, Varma R, Lawton F & Blackledge G (1994). Intervention debulking surgery in advanced epithelial ovarian cancer. *British Journal of Obstetrics and Gynaecology* **101**, 142–6.

Ripamonti C (1994). Management of bowel obstruction in advanced cancer. *Current Opinion in Oncology* **6**, 351–7.

Rodriguez M, Nguyen H, Averette H et al. (1994). National survey of ovarian carcinoma XII. Epithelial ovarian malignancies in women less than or equal to 25 years of age. *Cancer* 73(**4**), 1245–50.

Rubin S C, Hoskins W J, Benjamin I & Lewis J L Jr (1989). Palliative surgery for intestinal obstruction in advanced ovarian cancer. *Gynecologic Oncology* **34**, 16–19.

Scarabelli C, Gallo A, Zarrelli A, Visentin C & Campagnutta E (1995). Systematic pelvic and para-aortic lymphadenectomy during cytoreductive surgery in advanced ovarian cancer: potential benefit on survival. *Gynecologic Oncology* 56(**3**), 328–37.

Schwartz P E & Smith J P (1980). Second look operations in ovarian cancer. *American Journal of Obstetrics and Gynaecology* **138**, 1124–30.

Segna R, Dottino P, Mandeli J, Konsker K & Cohen C (1993). Secondary cytoreduction for ovarian cancer following cisplatin therapy. *Journal of Clinical Oncology* 11(**3**), 434–9.

Skipper H (1983). Stepwise progress in the treatment of disseminated cancers. *Cancer* **5**, 1773–9.

Surwit E, Childers J, Atlas I et al. (1996). Neoadjuvant chemotherapy for advanced ovarian cancer. *International Journal of Gynecologic Cancer* **6**, 356–61.

Trimble E L & Trimble C L (1993). Epithelial ovarian tumours of low malignant potential. In *Cancer of the ovary* (ed. M Markman & W J Hoskins), p.415. Raven Press, New York.

Tunca J C, Buchler D A, Mack E A, Ruzicka F F, Crowley J J & Carr W F (1981). The management of ovarian cancer-caused bowel obstruction. *Gynecologic Oncology* **12**, 186–92.

Unzelman R (1992). Advanced epithelial ovarian carcinoma: long-term survival experience at the community hospital. *American Journal of Obstetrics and Gynaecology* **166**, 1663–71.

van der Burg MEL, van Lent M, Buyse M et al. (1995). The effect of debulking surgery after induction chemotherapy on the prognosis in advanced epithelial ovarian cancer. *New England Journal of Medicine* **332**, 629–34.

Wharton J & Herson J (1981). Surgery for common epithelial tumours of the ovary. *Cancer* **48**, 582–9.

Williams S, Wong L C & Ngan H Y S (1998). Management of ovarian germ cell tumours. In *Ovarian cancer: controversies in management* (ed. D M Gershenson & W P MacGuire), pp.399–415. Churchill Livingstone, Edinburgh.

Wiltshaw E, Shepherd J H & Crowther M (1987). Salvage surgery – results. In *Ovarian cancer – the way ahead* (ed. W P Mason & F Sharp), pp.313–18. RCOG, London.

Chapter 8

The evidence base for medical intervention in ovarian cancer

Martin Gore

Introduction

The two most important and consistently defined prognostic factors in epithelial ovarian cancer are FIGO stage at diagnosis and the size of residual disease after initial surgery. Patients with early-stage ovarian cancer are those with disease confined to one or both ovaries (stage I); these patients have a good prognosis with five-year survival rate exceeding 80 per cent. The prognosis of patients with advanced disease, where the tumour has spread within the abdominal cavity, have a significantly worse prognosis with only 20 per cent of patients surviving five years (Friedlander 1998). The reason why overall survival in ovarian cancer is so poor (five-year survival 30 per cent) is that the majority of patients (70–80 per cent) present with advanced disease (Pettersson 1998).

Residual disease after surgery is the second most important factor that defines prognosis and this is described in virtually every multivariate analysis for prognostic factors that appears in the literature. Residual disease is a continuous variable but many investigators now use a cut-off dimension of 1 cm to define whether patients have been optimally or suboptimally debulked and thus have a good or a bad prognosis. The percentage of patients surviving three years is approximately 75, 50 and 25 per cent for those with no macroscopic residuum, residuum of ≤ 1 cm and >5 cm, respectively (Neijt 1991).

Prognostic factors, including those described above, allow a subpopulation of potentially curable patients to be identified and it is particularly important that these patients should receive optimum therapy with curative intent. Other parameters that have been shown in some multivariate analyses to be of prognostic significance include age of the patient, histology, performance status, ploidy and grade of tumour (Friedlander 1998).

It is becoming increasingly evident that patients do better when managed within the context of multidisciplinary teams whose personnel include doctors, nurses and associated health care professionals who have expertise in a particular type of cancer and are treatment-related specialists, i.e. surgery should be performed by gynaecological oncologists, radiotherapy should be supervised by radiotherapists specifically trained in the techniques of pelvic radiotherapy, and nurses should ideally have both oncological and gynaecological expertise (Junor *et al.* 1994). There is now widespread acceptance of the 'cancer centre/unit' configuration of UK cancer services, as recommended in the Calman/Hine report (Department of Health 1995), and this structure should help to encourage both site and modality specialisation for all cancers, not just gynaecological malignancy.

The main issues in chemotherapy for epithelial ovarian cancer are:

- should all patients receive adjuvant chemotherapy?
- should all patients receive platinum-based chemotherapy?
- is combination chemotherapy superior to single-agent treatment?
- is there a role for dose intensity?
- what is the role of paclitaxel?
- how should relapsed/refractory disease be managed?

These are examined below.

Should all patients receive adjuvant chemotherapy?

It is widely accepted that all patients with advanced disease (stage II–IV) should receive adjuvant chemotherapy, as the relapse rate following surgery without any further treatment approaches 100 per cent. There are no contemporary randomised data on which to base the overall survival benefit obtained from adjuvant chemotherapy; the benefit is assumed from the results of recent randomised studies where one treatment is shown to be superior to another.

Not all patients with ovarian cancer require chemotherapy following surgery. Patients with stage Ia or Ib disease with well- or moderately-differentiated tumours have an excellent five-year survival of approximately 80–90 per cent and there are no randomised data to suggest that adjuvant chemotherapy is of benefit (Ahmed *et al.* 1996; Friedlander 1998). Other substages of epithelial ovarian cancer, i.e. Ic disease, clear cell histology or those with poorly differentiated tumours have a higher relapse rate, in the order of 30–40 per cent, and these patients are often considered for chemotherapy (Ahmed et al. 1996). There are no randomised data that show a survival benefit for treating this group of patients, the recommendation for adjuvant chemotherapy is made on the inference that the best regimen for more-advanced cases is likely to have an even greater effect on lower stages of disease. It is always assumed that chemotherapy has its greatest effect on minimal residual disease.

There are three randomised trials currently taking place that are designed to resolve the issue of adjuvant chemotherapy in early-stage disease (MRC, ACTION, NOCOVA). In these trials patients who, as we have described above, are at high risk of relapse, are randomised to receive platinum-based chemotherapy or observation only. The number of events in such studies is small because of the good prognosis of the patient population and therefore very large numbers are needed to demonstrate a benefit for chemotherapy. It is unlikely that any of these trials are individually going to show a significant survival benefit for treatment and it is probable that a meta-analysis will have to be performed in order to resolve this issue. These trials were initiated while there was still some debate as to whether or not single-agent carboplatin or combination platinum-based therapy was standard treatment, and before the introduction of paclitaxel. Interpretation in the light of modern standard chemotherapy may therefore be difficult. We may need to make inferences from data obtained from advanced disease trials with regard to the gold standard therapy in this group of patients, as repeating these studies may be difficult.

Should all patients receive platinum-based chemotherapy?

Standard therapy for ovarian cancer originally involved the use of alkylating agents and a number of trials compared the use of combination chemotherapy to single-agent treatment (Advanced Ovarian Cancer Trialists Group 1991). Cisplatin was developed for ovarian cancer in the mid-1970s as a result of a relatively high response rate being observed (27 per cent) in previously treated patients (Wiltshaw & Carr 1974). Cisplatin was compared to alkylating agent therapy in a series of randomised trials and was shown to be superior in terms of remission rates, with overall responses in the range of 50–60 per cent as opposed to 30–40 per cent. In addition, about 20–25 per cent patients treated with cisplatin achieved a complete remission. Progression-free survival was also superior in most of the randomised studies but virtually all randomised studies failed to show an overall survival benefit (Advanced Ovarian Cancer Trialists Group 1991). The reason for this was that the randomised studies were not true comparisons of cisplatin versus alkylating agents but rather comparisons of alkylating agents followed by cisplatin versus cisplatin followed by alkylating agents. Cisplatin is more active in terms of response rate than alkylating agents and thus patients in the alkylating agent arms were being effectively 'rescued' by subsequent cisplatin therapy. This crossing over to cisplatin treatment is specifically noted in many of the trial reports. Nevertheless, cisplatin became standard therapy for ovarian cancer because of the highly statistically significant benefit that it conferred in relation to response rates and progression-free survival (Allen *et al.* 1993). In addition, two population-based studies have shown that despite the lack of overall survival benefit seen in the randomised trials or indeed in the original Ovarian Cancer Trialists Group's meta-analysis, population-based data demonstrate very clear, highly statistically significant survival benefits for the use of platinum compounds (Hunter *et al.* 1992; Junor *et al.* 1994).

One of the problems that surrounded the early introduction of cisplatin into general oncological practice was the toxicity of the compound. In particular, cisplatin-induced nausea and vomiting were very difficult to deal with, and it was not until the development of combination anti-emetic regimens, including the use of chlorpromazine, standard or high-dose metoclopramide, steroids and benzodiazepines, that cisplatin could start to be delivered in most units. Subsequently, in the mid-late 1980s the development of 5HT3 antagonists was a further step in improving the ease of delivery of this otherwise toxic compound.

In the early 1980s Harrap, Calvert and Wiltshaw at the Institute of Cancer Research and Royal Marsden Hospital (Calvert *et al.* 1985; Evans *et al.* 1998) developed carboplatin, which is an analogue of cisplatin. Carboplatin was quickly shown to be significantly less toxic than the parent compound, with less nausea and vomiting and, at standard doses, virtually no oto-, neuro- or nephro-toxicity. There was, however, more myelosuppression, mainly thrombocytopenia but this was not clinically significant at standard doses. The later development of dosing schedules by Calvert and colleagues that involved calculating the dose according to the glomerular filtration rate rather than the surface area of the patient further improved the safety of carboplatin because the dosing formula could accurately predict for the degree of thrombocytopenia (Calvert *et al.* 1989). Even when carboplatin was delivered at high doses, the drug was very well tolerated (Gore *et al.* 1987).

Randomised trials comparing single-agent cisplatin and carboplatin showed that there was little to choose between the two drugs in terms of overall response rates, progression-free survival or overall survival and this has been confirmed by a meta-analysis (Advanced Ovarian Cancer Trialists Group 1998). Nevertheless, there is still some controversy surrounding the substitution of carboplatin for cisplatin in that subgroup of patients who are potentially curable by chemotherapy. Some have argued that even if there is a small decrement in the order of 3 per cent in overall survival, this does not justify using carboplatin. Others feel that the difference in toxicity is such that small decrements in survival can be justified. The controversy concerning the use of carboplatin in potentially curable patients is very current within the context of platinum-paclitaxel therapy, and this will be discussed in a later section.

Is combination chemotherapy superior to single-agent treatment?

Once the use of platinum-based chemotherapy was established in the 1980s, the next issue concerned the use of platinum-based combination therapy. The commonest drugs used with platinum in such combinations were alkylating agents, anthracyclines, hexamethylmelamine and, occasionally, 5-FU. Platinum-based combinations were undoubtedly more toxic than single-agent therapy, particularly with regard to myelosuppression and, although generally response rates in randomised trials appeared higher than for single-agent platinum, approximately 70–80 per cent, most trials failed to show an improvement in overall survival (Advanced Ovarian Cancer Trialists Group 1991). A number, however, showed a difference in progression-free survival.

The discussions concerning the use of single-agent therapy were particularly polarised because single-agent carboplatin quickly came to be the preferred single-agent platinum therapy of choice. The therapeutic index for this compound was so much higher than combination therapy, particularly if cisplatin was used in the combination, that in many parts of Europe, including the UK, single-agent carboplatin was standard treatment. Even when a meta-analysis in 1991 (Advanced Ovarian Cancer Trialists Group 1991) showed a small but statistically significant (p=0.03) benefit for combination therapy, single-agent carboplatin remained standard therapy in the UK because of its toxicity profile. Some specialists took a pragmatic approach to this problem and felt that, for potentially curable patients, platinum-based combinations should be used, but for incurable patients (i.e. bulky stage III, stage IV, the elderly and frail) single-agent carboplatin was good and effective palliative chemotherapy.

Is there a role for dose intensity?

An important concept in solid tumour chemotherapy concerns the concentration of cytotoxics delivered to a tumour because *in vitro* data suggest that in some circumstances, drug resistance can be overcome by increasing the dose of drug delivered to the tumour cell (Griswold *et al.* 1987). In clinical practice, increasing the dose and/or intensity of chemotherapy may enhance the effectiveness of treatment. This is the rationale for high-dose chemotherapy regimens, which in randomised trials have shown to be effective treatments in haematological malignancies. The role of high-dose or intensive treatment in solid tumour oncology remains to be established but it is an area of active investigation in most tumour types, including epithelial ovarian cancer.

The methods of increasing dose intensity include increasing the number of cycles of treatment, the delivery of high-dose chemotherapy with bone marrow or peripheral blood stem cell rescue, or increasing the dose of drug in the standard treatment cycles. In epithelial ovarian cancer a further method of increasing dose intensity is available to the investigator – namely, intraperitoneal treatment. This is a rational route of administration in this disease because it is confined to the peritoneal cavity for a large part of its natural history. To date, the majority of studies investigating these different methods of dose intensity have focused on attempting to deliver more elemental platinum to the tumour.

There are over 40 reports of 27 different high-dose regimens in the literature with most studies involving small numbers of patients (Gore 1998a). No conclusions can be drawn from these data but there are currently two randomised trials in progress examining this question. By contrast, there are at least ten published randomised trials of dose intensity (Ngan *et al.* 1989; Colombo *et al.* 1993; Murphy *et al.* 1993; Bella *et al.* 1994; McGuire *et al.* 1995; Conte *et al.* 1996; Dittrich *et al.* 1996; Kaye *et al.* 1996; Jacobsen *et al.* 1997; Gore *et al.* 1998). All these trials examined increasing the dose intensity of platinum but then only by a factor of 2. Two of the smaller trials (Ngan *et al.* 1989; Bella *et al.* 1994) suggested a benefit but all the rest showed no increase in survival for more aggressive treatment. One of the main problems in dose-intensifying cisplatin is that it is impossible to deliver more than six cycles of cisplatin at 100 mg/m^2 without very significant toxicity, and this has been a particular feature of the trials that have involved this drug. Thus, on the current evidence from randomised clinical trials, there appears to be no place for increasing the dose and/or the intensity of platinum in standard regimens for ovarian cancer outside the context of a clinical trial; furthermore, increments of two-fold are of no benefit.

Intraperitoneal therapy is an opportunity to increase the concentration of cytotoxic agents in close proximity to tumour deposits since they are scattered throughout the peritoneum in advanced disease. The concentration of platinum compounds in peritoneal fluid can be increased by 20- or 30-fold by their intraperitoneal delivery, although this is not always translated into a pharmacological advantage in terms of area under the concentration time curve (Markman 1993). However, chemotherapy does not penetrate beyond 2–3 mm of the tumour nodule and data in the late 1980s (Howell *et al.* 1997) demonstrated in non-randomised studies that there was no benefit to intraperitoneal therapy if patients had peritoneal nodules bigger than 2 cm. This was subsequently confirmed in a multivariate analysis of data derived from non-randomised phase II trials (Markman 1993).

Until 1996 there were no randomised data to support the use of intraperitoneal chemotherapy either as first-line treatment or in the relapsed setting. However, Alberts *et al.* (1996) demonstrated that for patients with optimally debulked disease (<1 cm residuum) there was a statistically significant survival benefit for those patients who had cisplatin delivered intraperitoneally as compared to the intravenous route. Patients who received intraperitoneal cisplatin experienced less severe platinum-related side-effects such as oto-, neuro- and nephro-toxicity. The problems with this study included the length of time it took to accrue patients and the considerable efforts that were required to standardise intraperitoneal catheter placement and care.

Recently, the Gynecologic Oncology Group (GOG) have presented data from a second randomised trial involving patients with optimally debulked disease where one arm included cisplatin delivered intraperitoneally (Markham *et al.* 1998).

Patients were randomised to receive intravenous cisplatin and paclitaxel or two cycles of high-dose carboplatin intravenously followed by intravenous paclitaxel and intraperitoneal cisplatin. There was a statistically significant progression-free survival advantage for patients treated with intraperitoneal cisplatin but no overall survival advantage. One of the problems with this trial was that nearly 10 per cent patients randomised to intraperitoneal cisplatin never received this treatment and this was thought to be due to the cumulative toxicity of the previously delivered high-dose carboplatin. It is interesting to observe the discussion among experts in the field when these data were presented; exponents of the intraperitoneal route cite the results to support the use of intraperitoneal therapy, whereas those who are sceptical of its use, point out that no overall survival advantage was demonstrated in this trial.

Intraperitoneal chemotherapy has the potential of causing a number of problems, including peritonitis, adhesion formation, loculation of fluid and intestinal obstruction. Many feel that these potential side-effects render this route of administration impractical, whereas other claim that with careful attention to detail and good education the complication rate can be minimised. There are additional problems, including the difficulty of ensuring an even distribution of the cytotoxic agent throughout all surfaces of the peritoneal cavity, as well as doubts concerning the true pharmacodynamic advantage of this route of administration.

This author's view is that the two randomised studies that have been reported suggest it is reasonable to continue to investigate the use of intraperitoneal therapy within the context of clinical trials. However, in view of the practical problems associated with the intraperitoneal route and the recent development of a new gold standard of intravenous therapy, the use of intraperitoneal therapy outside of a trial cannot yet be advocated. Further studies are required that compare this route of administration with new standard intravenous regimens.

What is the role of paclitaxel?

In the early 1990s phase II trials in patients with relapsed and refractory epithelial ovarian cancer suggested that a new class of compound, the taxanes, was active. Initial response rates suggested that approximately 30 per cent of patients with relapsed/refractory ovarian cancer would respond to paclitaxel, although subsequent phase II studies suggested that the response rate in this patient population was lower, 15–20 per cent (McGuire *et al.* 1989; Einzig *et al.* 1992; Thigpen *et al.* 1994; Gore 1996). The activity of paclitaxel in relapsed/refractory disease led to the initiation of trials where paclitaxel was given as part of first-line therapy.

The first such trial was initiated by the GOG and reported in 1996 (McGuire *et al.* 1996). Patients with suboptimally debulked advanced disease were randomised to receive cisplatin plus cyclophosphamide or cisplatin plus paclitaxel. Paclitaxel was given at a dose of 135 mg/m^2 over 24 hours and treatment was cycled every 21 days. There was a significant benefit in terms of response rate, progression-free survival and overall survival for patients treated with cisplatin-paclitaxel. The improvement in median survival was 14 months and the regimen immediately became standard therapy in the USA. In Europe most investigators felt that a confirmatory trial was required because standard therapy should not be changed simply as the result of one study, particularly when the new therapy was significantly more expensive than current standard practice. In addition, there was a counterintuitive result within the data because the improvement in progression-free survival, although significant, was less than the improvement in overall survival, a result which is rather unusual.

An intergroup involving the EORTC, NCIC, Scottish Co-operative Group and the Scandinavian Co-operative Group has now presented the results of a confirmatory study (Stuart *et al.* 1998). In this study both optimally and suboptimally debulked patients were randomised and in the experimental arm, paclitaxel was given at 175 mg/m^2 over three hours. This trial has almost exactly repeated the results published by the GOG with a highly statistically significant improvement in overall survival of about one year. When these two trials are analysed together, the survival advantage for patients treated with cisplatin-paclitaxel as opposed to cisplatin-cyclophosphamide is hugely significant (p=0.000001) (Adams *et al.* 1998). The main problem with the intergroup study has been a high degree of grade 3/4 neurotoxicity seen with the three-hour schedule, and this is much greater than that reported when paclitaxel is delivered at 135 mg/m^2 over 24 hours.

A third study that has reported its results (Muggia *et al.* 1997) involved randomising patients to either single-agent paclitaxel or single-agent cisplatin or a combination of the two. There were no survival differences between the three arms of the study but the crossover rate between cisplatin and paclitaxel in the single-agent arms was very high and indeed a number of patients (almost 50 per cent) received alternative therapy before progression was defined. Thus, the study is really a trial of sequential platinum-paclitaxel. The problem of interpreting these data is reminiscent of the difficulties encountered with the early survival data from the platinum versus non-platinum trials in the 1970s and 1980s where crossover therapy confounded the analyses.

Pre-paclitaxel, as has already been mentioned, the suggestion had been that carboplatin could be substituted for cisplatin. There is no disagreement among experts in the field that platinum-paclitaxel is standard therapy for ovarian cancer but there is considerable disagreement over whether carboplatin can be substituted for cisplatin in all circumstances. The same arguments as have previously been described apply within the context of paclitaxel therapy – namely, whether or not this substitution can be made in patients who are potentially curable. Carboplatin plus paclitaxel is a well-tolerated regimen and it is undoubtedly the best palliative first-line therapy. There are three trials which will answer the question as to whether or not it is safe to use carboplatin instead of cisplatin within the context of potentially curable patients. Data from these trials (Neijt *et al.* 1997; du Bois *et al.* 1998; Ozols *et al.* 1999) suggest that there is little to choose between cisplatin-paclitaxel and carboplatin-paclitaxel in terms of response rates and progression-free and overall survival.

A MRC trial (ICON 3) closed to accrual in 1998. This study randomised patients to receive either carboplatin-paclitaxel or control treatments which could be either carboplatin or cisplatin-adriamycin-cyclophosphamide, according to investigator discretion. This was a very large trial, with approximately 2,000 patients, and will be the only comparison of carboplatin-paclitaxel against non-paclitaxel containing chemotherapy.

How should relapsed/refractory disease be managed?

Patients with relapsed epithelial ovarian cancer are incurable. Chemotherapy for these women must be viewed as palliative and therefore the toxicity of treatment is a very important consideration. The likelihood of a response to second-line treatment is dependent on a number of factors that have been defined in non-randomised trials and include the length of time between initial treatment to the start of second-line therapy, the bulk of disease, the number of sites of disease, previous response, histology and the absence of anaemia (Eisenhauer *et al.* 1997). Patients who relapse with a disease-free interval of longer than one year have a good chance of responding again to platinum-based chemotherapy, whereas patients who relapse soon after first-line therapy are unlikely to benefit from further platinum (Gore *et al.* 1990; Markham *et al.* 1991). Failing one platinum compound usually means resistance to another (Taylor *et al.* 1994; Gore *et al.* 1995). Thus, patients who relapse within one year are frequently entered into phase II trials and, interestingly, the new compounds that have been studied in this patient population over the last three years (i.e. topotecan, hexalen, liposomal doxorubicin and gemcitabine) have all given similar response rates of approximately 20 per cent (Gore 1998b).

There are few randomised trials in patients with relapsed disease and most compare two treatments; there are no trials of chemotherapy versus best supportive care. Nevertheless, the randomised trials that there have been provide useful data; for instance, a randomised trial comparing topotecan with paclitaxel in the relapsed setting (ten Bokkel Huinink *et al.* 1997) showed that both compounds have very similar activity and that response rates are lower within the context of this randomised trial than in previous single-arm phase II studies. Combination therapies, including etoposide and cisplatin or epirubicin, cisplatin and infusional 5-FU, have shown high response rates in patients who relapse within 12 months but these combinations are associated with more toxicity (Ahmed *et al.* 1995; van der Burg *et al.* 1996). A randomised trial that compared single-agent paclitaxel with combination platinum-based chemotherapy in patients who had relapsed over one year (Bolis *et al.* 1996) showed there was a clear advantage in terms of response rate to the platinum-based combination.

At the present time patients with relapsed disease should be offered palliative chemotherapy but, where possible, they should be entered into clinical trials. Patients who relapse with a disease-free interval of greater than one year should, at some stage, receive further platinum therapy and patients with truly refractory disease probably should not receive more than two lines of treatment, as they are unlikely to benefit from repeated treatments with different drugs. A particularly difficult management problem is the timing of second-line treatment and whether this should be started at the first sign of relapse (e.g. a rising CA 125 with no macroscopic evidence of disease on CT scan) or whether one should wait for measurable progression with or without symptoms. An important randomised trial is being conducted by the MRC in this patient population; patients are randomised to receive treatment on a rising CA 125 or no treatment until macroscopic evidence of disease and/or symptoms. In the meantime, this author's policy is not to treat patients on a rising CA 125 alone but, in view of the data from Eisenhauer *et al.* (1997), one should probably treat patients before the disease gets very bulky (i.e. >5 cm).

Palliation

The main symptoms suffered by patients with ovarian cancer are recurrent ascites, abdominal pain, usually associated with subacute intestinal obstruction, and intestinal obstruction itself with its associated symptoms of vomiting and constipation. Patients who respond to chemotherapy are likely to have these symptoms palliated and therefore the decision to use chemotherapy to palliate these symptoms is based on the likelihood of a response. In general, chemotherapy does not palliate patients with intestinal obstruction and is rarely used, except when there is intestinal obstruction at presentation and patients are chemonaive.

A number of methods have been used to palliate ascites, including repeated paracentesis, Levine shunts, diuretics and physical methods such as binding and exercises. None of these methods has been tested in a randomised fashion and treatment tends to be individualised.

An extensive systematic review of the literature on the palliation of intestinal obstruction in patients with advanced gynaecological and intestinal malignancy (Feuer *et al.* 1998) examined the use of corticosteroids, anti-emetics, analgesics, somatostatin, surgery, gastrotomy tubes, chemotherapy, radiotherapy and total parenteral nutrition. The evidence base for these interventions was poor in terms of prospective randomised clinical trials, although many uncontrolled retrospective series have examined the use of all these modalities in the management of intestinal obstruction.

There are two randomised trials of the use of corticosteroids in bowel obstruction due to gynaecological and GI malignancy (Hardy *et al.* 1999; Laval *et al.* 1998) and although there is a suggestion that patients treated with steroids benefited, the number of patients involved is too small to make any firm conclusions. There are no randomised trials investigating the role of anti-emetics, analgesics, somatostatin or analogues, surgery, chemotherapy, radiotherapy or total parenteral nutrition. There is, however, one randomised trial of percutaneous endoscopic gastrostomy (Cannizzaro *et al.* 1995) but this compared two different gauges of catheter rather than the insertion of a catheter versus best supportive care.

Conclusions

The evidence base for medical intervention in ovarian cancer clearly shows that a combination of platinum and paclitaxel is standard treatment for those requiring first-line chemotherapy. Patients with advanced disease (stage II, III, IV) require such treatment, whereas patients with good-prognosis early-disease do not (stage Ia or Ib, grade 1 or 2). There is a grey area between these two patient groups where there is considerable uncertainty as to whether or not patients benefit from adjuvant chemotherapy after surgery; the results of three current randomised trials in this patient population are awaited. There was controversy over whether or not carboplatin can be substituted for cisplatin in the context of first-line paclitaxel-platinum combination therapy. This substitution is now reasonable in the light of recently presented data from randomised trials comparing cisplatin-paclitaxel with carboplatin-paclitaxel.

References

Adams M, A'Hern R P, Calvert A H *et al.* (1998). Chemotherapy for ovarian cancer. A consensus statement on standard practice. *Br J Cancer* **78**, 1404–6.

Advanced Ovarian Cancer Trialists Group (1991). Chemotherapy in advanced ovarian cancer: an overview of randomised clinical trials. *Br Med J* **303**, 884–93.

Advanced Ovarian Cancer Trialists Group (1998). Chemotherapy in advanced ovarian cancer: four systematic meta-analyses of individual patient data from thirty-seven randomised trials. *Br J Cancer* **78**, 1479–87.

Ahmed F, Kinf D M, Nicol B *et al.* (1995). Preliminary results of infusional chemotherapy (cisplatin, epirubicin and 5-fluorouracil, ECF) for refractory and relapsed epithelial ovarian cancer. *Proc Am Soc Clin Oncol* **14**, 790.

Ahmed F Y, Wiltshaw E, A'Hern R P *et al.* (1996). Natural history and prognosis of untreated stage I epithelial ovarian carcinoma. *J Clin Oncol* **14**(11), 2968–75.

Alberts D S, Liu P Y, Hannigan E V *et al.* (1996). Intraperitoneal cisplatin plus intravenous cyclophosphamide versus intravenous cisplatin plus intravenous cyclophosphamide for stage III ovarian cancer [see comments]. *N Engl J Med* **335**(26), 1950–5.

Allen D G, Baak J, Belpomme D *et al.* (1993). Advanced epithelial ovarian cancer: 1993 consensus statements. *Ann Oncol* **4** (Suppl.4), S83–8.

Bella M, Cocconi G, Lotticci R *et al.* (1994). Mature results of a prospective randomised trial comparing two different dose-intensity regimens of cisplatin in advanced ovarian carcinoma. *Ann Oncol* **5** (Suppl.8), S23.

Bolis G, Scarfone G, Villa A *et al.* (1996). A randomised study in recurrent ovarian cancer comparing the efficacy of single agent versus combination chemotherapy, according to time to relapse. *Proc Am Soc Clin Oncol* **15**, 750.

Calvert A H, Harland S J, Newell D R *et al.* (1985). Phase I studies with carboplatin at the Royal Marsden Hospital. *Cancer Treatment Reviews* **12** (Suppl.A), 51–7.

Calvert A H, Newell D R, Gumbrell L A *et al.* (1989). Carboplatin dosage: prospective evaluation of a simple formula based on renal function. *J Clin Oncol* **7**, 1748.

Cannizzaro R, Bortoluzzi F, Valentini M *et al.* (1995). Percutaneous endoscopic gastrostomy as a decompressive technique in bowel obstruction due to abdominal carcinomatosis. *Endoscopy* **27**, 317–20.

Colombo N, Pittelli M R & Parma G (1993). Cisplatin (P) dose intensity in advanced ovarian cancer (AOC): a randomised study of conventional dose (DC) vs dose-intense (DI) cisplatin monochemotherapy. *Proc Am Soc Clin Oncol* **12**, 255.

Conte P F, Bruzzone M, Carnino F *et al.* (1996). High-dose versus low-dose cisplatin in combination with cyclophosphamide and epidoxorubicin in suboptimal ovarian cancer: a randomised study of the Gruppo Oncologico Nord-Ovest. *J Clin Onc* **14** 351–6.

Department of Health (1995). *A policy framework for commissioning cancer services: a report of the Expert Advisory Group on Cancer to the Chief Medical Officers of England and Wales.* HM Stationery Office, London.

Dittrich C, Obermair A, Kurz C *et al.* (1996). Prospective randomised trial of cisplatin/carboplatin versus conventional cisplatin/cyclophosphamide in epithelial ovarian cancer: first results of the impact of platinum dose intensity on patient outcome. *Proc Am Soc Clin Oncol* **15**, 749.

du Bois A, Lueck H J, Meier W, Moebus V, Costa S D, Bauknecht T *et al.* (1999). Cisplatin/paclitaxel versus carboplatin/paclitaxel in ovarian cancer: update of an Arbeitsgemeinschaft Gynaecologiske Onkologie (AGO) Study Group Trial. *Proc Am Soc Clin Oncol* **18**, 1374.

Einzig AI, Wiernik P H, Sasloff J *et al.* (1992). Phase II study and long-term follow up of patients treated with taxol for advanced ovarian adenocarcinoma. *J Clin Oncol* **10**, 1748–53.

Eisenhauer E A, Vermorken J B & Van Glabbeke M (1997). Predictors of response to subsequent chemotherapy in platinum-pretreated ovarian cancer. *Ann Oncol* **8**(10), 963–8.

Evans B D, Chapman P, Dady P *et al.* (1998). A phase II study of carboplatin and chlorambucil in previously untreated patients with advanced ovarian cancer. *ASCO* **7**, A536.

Feuer D J, Brodley K E & Tate A T (1998). *Systematic review of the management of intestinal obstruction due to advanced gynaecological and intestinal cancer.* NHS Executive Research and Development Project NCP 2/1211.

Friedlander M (1998). Prognostic factors. In *Ovarian cancer 5* (ed. F Sharp, T Blackett, J Berek & R Bast), pp.199–216. Isis Medical Media, Oxford.

Gore M E (1996). The role of taxanes. In *Ovarian cancer 4* (ed. F Sharp, T Blackett, R Leake & J Berek) pp.143–52. Chapman and Hall Medical, London.

Gore M E (1998a). Overview – high dose and intraperitoneal therapy. In *Ovarian cancer 5* (ed. F Sharp, T Blackett, J Berek & R Bast), pp.311–20. Isis Medical Media, Oxford.

Gore M E (1998b). Strategies for new drugs and their combination. In *Ovarian cancer 5* (ed. F Sharp, T Blackett, J Berek & R Bast), pp.363–72. Isis Medical Media, Oxford.

Gore M E, Calvert A H & Smith I E (1987). High dose carboplatin in the treatment of lung cancer and mesothelioma: a phase I dose escalation study. *Eur J Cancer Clin Oncol* **23**, 1391–7.

Gore M E, Fryatt I, Wiltshaw E *et al.* (1990). Treatment of relapsed ovary with cisplatin or carboplatin following initial treatment with these compounds. *Gynecol Oncol* **36**, 207–11.

Gore M E, Preston N, A'Hern R P *et al.* (1995). Platinum-taxol non-cross resistance in epithelial ovarian cancer. *Br J Cancer* **70**, 1308–10.

Gore M E, A'Hern R P & Swenerton K (1997). Good manners for the pharmaceutical industry. *Lancet* **350**, 370.

Gore M E, Mainwaring P N, A'Hern R P *et al.* (1998). Randomised trial of dose intensity with single agent carboplatin in patients with epithelial ovarian cancer. *J Clin Oncol* **16**, 2426–34.

Griswold D P, Trader M W, Freii E *et al.* (1987). Response of drug-sensitive and resistant L1210 leukemias to high-dose chemotherapy. *Cancer Res* **47**, 2323–7.

Hardy J R, Ling P J, Mansi J *et al.* (1999). Pitfalls in placebo controlled trials in palliative care: dexamethasone for the palliation of malignant bowel obstruction. *Palliative Medicine* (in press).

Howell S B, Zimm S, Markman M *et al.* (1997). Long-term survival of advanced refractory ovarian carcinoma patients with small-volume disease treated with intraperitoneal chemotherapy. *J Clin Oncol* **5**(10), 1607–12.

Hunter W E, Alexander N D E & Soutter W P (1996). Meta-analysis of surgery in advanced ovarian carcinoma: is maximum cytoreductive surgery an independent determinant of prognosis? *Am J Obstet Gynecol* **166**, 505–11.

Jackobsen A, Bertelsen K, Andersen J E *et al.* (1997). Dose-effect study of carboplatin in ovarian cancer. A Danish Ovarian Cancer Group Study. *J Clin Onc* **15**, 193.

Junor E J, Hole D J & Gillis C R (1994). Management of ovarian cancer: referral to a multidisciplinary team matters. *Br J Cancer* **70**(2), 363–70.

Kaye S B, Paul J, Cassidy J *et al.* (1996). Mature results of a randomised trial of two doses of cisplatin for the treatment of ovarian cancer. *J Clin Onc* **14**, 2113.

Laval G, Girardier J, Lassauniere JM *et al.* (1998). Multi-centre double-blind randomised clinical trial on the use of methylprednisolone in non-surgical cancer related bowel obstruction. (Personal communication)

McGuire W P, Rowinsky E K, Rosenhein N B *et al.* (1989). Taxol: a unique antineoplastic agent with significant activity in advanced ovarian epithelial neoplasms. *Ann Intern Med* **111**(4), 273–9.

McGuire W P, Hoskins W J, Bradey M F *et al.* (1995). Assessment of dose-intensive therapy in suboptimally debulked ovarian cancer: a Gynaecologic Oncology Group study. *J Clin Onc* **13**, 1589–99.

McGuire W P, Hoskins W J, Brady M F *et al.* (1996). Cyclophosphamide and cisplatin compared with paclitaxel and cisplatin in patients with stage III and stage IV ovarian cancer. *N Engl J Med* **334**(1), 1–6.

Markham M, Rothman R, Hakes T *et al.* (1991). Second-line platinum therapy in patients with ovarian cancer previously treated with cisplatin. *J Clin Oncol* **9**, 389–93

Markham M, Bundy B, Benda J *et al.* (1998). Randomised phase 3 study of intravenous (IV) cisplatin (cis)/paclitaxel (pac) versus moderately high dose IV carboplatin (carb) … *Proc Am Soc Clin Oncol* **17**, 1392.

Markman M (1993). Intraperitoneal chemotherapy. In *Cancer of the ovary* (ed. M Markman & W J Hoskins), p.317. Raven Press.

Muggia F M, Brady P S, Brady M F *et al.* (1997). Phase III of cisplatin or paclitaxel, versus their combination in suboptimal stage III and IV epithelial ovarian cancer: Gynaecologic Oncology Group study No.132. *Proc Am Soc Clin Oncol* **16**, A1257.

Murphy D, Crowther D, Renninson J *et al.* (1993). A randomised dose intensity study in ovarian carcinoma comparing chemotherapy given at four week intervals for six cycles with half dose chemotherapy given for twelve cycles. *Ann Oncol* **4**.

Neijt J P, ten Bokkell Huinink W W, van der Burg M E L *et al.* (1991). Long-term survival in ovarian cancer. *Eur J Cancer* **27**, 1367–72.

Neijt J P, Hansen M, Hansen S W *et al.* (1997). Randomised phase III study in previously untreated epithelial ovarian cancer FIGO stage IIB, IIC, III, IV, comparing paclitaxel-cisplatin and paclitaxel-carboplatin. *Proc Am Soc Clin Oncol* **16**, A1259.

Ngan HYS, Choo YC, Cheung M *et al.* (1989). A randomised study of high-dose versus low-dose cisplatin combined with cyclophosphamide in the treatment of advanced ovarian cancer. *Chemotherapy* **35**(3), 221–7.

Ozols R F, Bundy B N, Fowler J, Clarke-Pearson D, Mannel R, Hartenbach E M *et al.* (1999). Randomized phase II study of cisplatin (CIS)/paclitaxel (PAC) versus carboplatin (CARBO)/PAC in optimal stage III epithelial ovarian cancer (OC): a Gynaecologic Oncology Group Trial (GOG 158). *Proc Am Soc Clin Oncol* **18**, 1373.

Pettersson F (1988). *Annual report of the results of treatment in gynecologic cancer.* International Federation of Gynaecology and Obstetrics (FIGO), vol.20.

Stuart G, Bertelsen K, Mangioni C *et al.* (1998). Updated analysis shows a highly significant improved overall survival (OS) for cisplatin-paclitaxel as first-line treatment of advanced ovarian cancer. Mature results of the EORTC-GCCG, NOCOVA, NCIC CTG and Scottish Intergroup trial. *Proc Am Soc Clin Oncol* **17**, A1394.

Taylor A E, Wiltshaw E, Gore M E *et al.* (1994). Long-term follow up of the first randomised study of cisplatin versus carboplatin for advanced epithelial ovarian cancer. *J Clin Oncol* **12**(10), 2066–70.

ten Bokkel Huinink W, Gore M, Carmichael J *et al.* (1997). Topotecan versus paclitaxel for the treatment of recurrent epithelial ovarian cancer. *J Clin Oncol* **15**, 2183–93.

Thigpen T, Blessing J A, Ball H *et al.* (1994). Phase II trial of paclitaxel in patients with progressive ovarian carcinoma after platinum-based chemotherapy: a Gynecologic Oncology Group study. *J Clin Oncol* **12**,1748–53.

van der Burg M, Logmans A, de Wit R *et al.* (1996). *Proc Am Soc Clin Oncol* **15**, 772.

Wiltshaw E & Carr T (1974). Cis-platinum (II) diamminedichloride: clinical experience of the Royal Marsden Hospital and Institute of Cancer Research. *Recent Results Cancer Res* **48**, 178–82.

Chapter 9

Clinical outcomes in ovarian cancer: service organisation and survival in the UK

Elizabeth Junor

Introduction

Reported five-year survival rates for patients diagnosed with ovarian cancer in North America and in Europe vary from 43 to 22 per cent (Millet *et al.* 1993; The Eurocare Study 1995). Figures for Great Britain lie towards the lower end of this span: Scotland 28 per cent, and England and Wales 26 per cent.

Variations in outcome within geographical areas in the UK have been reported (Forman & Rider 1996), with one district of Yorkshire showing significantly improved five-year survival rates at 46 per cent. The West Midlands Cancer Registry (West Midlands Regional Health Authority 1995) reports five-year relative survival rates for two districts as being statistically significantly poorer than other districts in the West Midlands. The Information and Statistics Division of the Scottish Office has published data by health board (Clinical Outcome Indicators Working Group 1996) showing statistically significant improved outcome for one health board.

When data are based on large numbers of cases, then any variation in prognostic variables will tend to be smoothed out, but care with interpretation of data must still be taken. Case mix and referral patterns will influence outcome, therefore when examining treatment-related features which influence outcome, every effort should be made to adjust for known prognostic variables.

Survival is the most easily measured outcome and therefore forms the basis of the following discussion; however, quality of life is equally, if not more important, but as no population data exist, it will not be further considered in this chapter.

Surgical and post-surgical management

Within the UK, evidence exists to show that the following features of management contribute to improve survival outcome for patients with ovarian cancer:

- Surgical management:
  - surgery performed by gynaecologists when compared with general surgeons
  - surgery performed by specialist gynaecologists when compared with general gynaecologists.

- Post-surgical management:
  - referral to non-surgical oncologists
  - multidisciplinary team management
  - prescription of platinum chemotherapy.

Surgical management
Gynaecologists versus general surgeons

Three population-based studies have been carried out within the UK which have examined variation in outcome with reference to whether surgery was performed by gynaecologists or general surgeons. All three studies performed multivariate analysis adjusting for the well-recognised prognostic variables of age, stage, histology and tumour grade. One study also adjusted for the presence of ascites.

The West Midland Cancer Registry-based study (Kehoe *et al.* 1994) was of 1,184 surgically treated patients registered between 1985 and 1987 using data from the Cancer Registry. Both the North Western Regional Cancer Registry-based study (691 surgically treated patients between 1991 and 1992) (Woodman *et al.* 1997), and the Scottish National Cancer Registration-based study (432 surgically treated patients registered in 1987) (Junor *et al.* 1994) relied on data specifically extracted from case notes for the studies. Using Cox's proportional hazard method with general gynaecologists as the baseline of 1, all three studies demonstrated a greater than 30 per cent decrease in survival for patients operated on by general surgeons (see Table 9.1).

Table 9.1 Gynaecologists versus general surgeons

Reference	No.	Year	Gynaecologists RR	Surgeons RR	95% CI
Junor *et al.* (1994)	432	1987	1	1.37	(1.05–1.77)
Kehoe *et al.* (1994)	1184	1985–7	1	1.34	(1.05–1.71)
Woodman *et al.* (1997)	691	1991–2	1	1.58	(1.19–2.1)

Both the Scottish and North Western studies reported that general surgeons were less likely to perform total abdominal hysterectomy, bilateral salpingo-oophrectomy and omentectomy and more likely than gynaecologists to only perform a biopsy. In the West Midlands, general surgeons were likely to perform only an oophorectomy in stage I disease (35.6 versus 16.4 per cent). In stage III disease, TAH BSO was performed significantly more often by gynaecologists than by general surgeons (p< 0.05).

It has been known since 1975 that the volume of remaining tumour after laparotomy influences survival (Griffiths 1975). The Scottish study demonstrated that after adjustment for prognostic factors, the likelihood of less than 2 cm of tumour remaining when a surgeon operated was 80 per cent less than when the operation was performed by a gynaecologist (gynaecologist baseline 1, general surgeons RR 0.2 (95 per cent CI 0.1–0.6), p< 0.01). Further analysis (Junor *et al.* 1994) showed that the relatively poorer survival for patients operated on by general surgeons was due to their failure to remove tumour.

Number of operations performed

Conclusive evidence in favour of gynaecologists performing the surgery has been presented, but do 'surgeons' (either general or gynaecologist) who frequently operate on patients with ovarian cancer have better outcomes than those who infrequently operate on ovarian cancer patients?

Woodman *et al.* (1997) found no relationship between workload of gynaecologists and outcome after adjustment for prognostic variables. Similarly, Kehoe *et al.* (1994) found a wide variation between the number of operations being performed by any one individual surgeon (median 3, range 1–22) or gynaecologist (median 8, range 1–33), but could not demonstrate an association between survival and the number of operations performed by an individual. In Scotland, patients operated on by a surgeon performing greater numbers of operations showed a trend towards better survival, but this did not retain statistical significance after adjustment for prognostic variables (see Table 9.2) (Junor *et al.* 1996).

Table 9.2 Relationship between survival and the number of patients operated on by an individual

Operations per year	Patient numbers	5-year survival (unadjusted) (%)	RHR unadjusted	adjusted*
1	159	16	1	1
2–4	225	27	0.73**	0.94
>5	72	33	0.54***	0.74†

Notes: * adjusted for prognostic factors: age, stage, histology, differentiation, ascites
 **p<0.01 ***p<0.001 †p<0.1

[*Source:* Junor *et al.* (1996)]

Specialist gynaecologists versus general gynaecologists

If gynaecologists have improved outcome compared with general surgeons because they leave less tumour behind at laparotomy, could specialist oncological gynaecologists further improve survival?

This question was addressed in a second study carried out in Scotland examining all patients registered to the Scottish Cancer Registration Scheme in 1987, 1992, 1993 and 1994 who had surgical intervention (Junor *et al.* 1999). Surgeons were classified as general surgeons, general gynaecologists or specialist gynaecologists. Again Cox's proportional hazard model was used, adjusting for age, stage, histology, degree of differentiation and presence of ascites. Specialist gynaecologists tended to operate on more late-stage (III + IV) cases than general gynaecologists (70 versus 57 per cent). At two years, there was an overall significantly improved survival for patients operated on by specialist gynaecologists; however, by three years, a survival advantage could only be demonstrated for stage III patients. Forty-four per cent (830/1866) presented in stage III. The advantage for treatment by specialists was 25 per cent (baseline 1 for general gynaecologists, for specialist gynaecologists RR 0.75 (95 per cent CI 0.62–0.92)). It was recognised that post-surgical management may have contributed to this difference, but when prescription of platinum chemotherapy was included in the model, the hazard ratio changed little (RR 0.77 95 per cent CI 0.63–0.95).

Having demonstrated that the survival difference between general surgeons and gynaecologists in 1987 (Junor *et al.* 1994) was due to the variation in the volume of disease remaining, this factor was examined for gynaecologists versus specialist gynaecologists. Specialist gynaecologists successfully debulked 36.3 per cent of cases to less than 2 cm, compared with 28.7 per cent for general gynaecologists. In those patients with less than 2 cm of disease remaining post-operatively, there was no difference in survival between specialist and general gynaecological cases, suggesting that an operation performed to debulk the tumour in an adequate way was the appropriate treatment, whoever operated. In the group of stage III patients, where more than 2 cm of tumour remained (72.6 per cent of stage III), there was a clear difference in survival (RR 0.71) for specialist gynaecologists. It is interesting to note that this group in which the greatest benefit was seen for specialist gynaecologists was the largest individual group but it is more difficult to interpret to what the benefit was due. There was no proof, but the authors consider that it is perhaps in the most surgically demanding cases, where the expertise of specialists is beneficial. It may be that a greater volume of tumour was removed, although still leaving behind disease classified as greater than 2 cm. No one believes that there is a magical cut-off at 1 cm, 2 cm or any other volume. Undoubtedly, the more tumour which is removed, one would anticipate, the better chance of further tumour reduction by chemotherapy.

An interesting geographical variation was found by health board with regard to specialist gynaecologists. It was evident that five health boards had more than 24 per cent (24–42 per cent) of patients operated on by specialists, while the remaining health boards had fewer than 5 per cent operated on by specialists. After adjusting for age, stage, histology, degree of differentiation and presence of ascites, the five 'high-usage' health boards were compared as a group with the remaining 'low-usage' health boards as a group. The 'high-usage' health boards performed significantly better at three years with a hazard ratio of 0.82 (95 per cent CI 0.73–0.92) against baseline 1 of the 'low-usage' health boards. It would also appear that those patients managed by general gynaecologists in the 'high-usage' health boards had an advantage over patients in the 'low-usage' health boards managed by general gynaecologists. Perhaps specialist gynaecologists influenced their non-specialist colleagues by dissemination of information, advice or some other unknown feature of management.

Post-surgical referral

Surgery is undoubtedly a major part of the management of patients with ovarian carcinoma. Likewise, the prescription of chemotherapy is accepted as a major contributing factor to improved outcome in ovarian cancer. The overview published by the Advanced Ovarian Cancer Trialists Group (1991) has shown the benefit of platinum chemotherapy and more recently, two major studies (McGuire *et al.* 1996; Stuart *et al.* 1998) have demonstrated, not only improved response rates, but improved disease-free survival by use of paclitaxel in combination with platinum compared with platinum in combination with cyclophosphamide.

There are no published data to suggest who should prescribe or deliver chemotherapy, but the population-based study from the North Western Regional Cancer Registry (Kehoe *et al.* 1994) has demonstrated a 46 per cent improved survival for patients referred to a non-surgical oncologist (RR 0.54 95 per cent CI 0.43–0.68). This study did not present data on the frequency or type of chemotherapy so it is not possible to determine which feature of management was contributed by the non-surgical oncologists, although it is likely that chemotherapy is a possibility. It is a matter of concern that in this study spanning patients diagnosed between 1991 and 1992, 47 per cent of patients were not referred to a non-surgical oncologist.

Multidisciplinary management

If referral to a non-surgical oncologist, which necessarily means involvement of another clinical discipline, improved survival, then could management by a team which includes not only gynaecologists with a special interest in malignancy but also non-surgical oncologists with a special interest in gynaecological malignancy, further improve outcome?

Returning again to the Scottish study of 1987 (Junor *et al.* 1994), management by a multidisciplinary team post-surgery was shown to be a highly significant (p 0.001) positive feature after adjustment for prognostic variables. As anticipated, patients referred to such joint management clinics were more likely to receive platinum chemotherapy (59.2 per cent) compared with those who were not referred (21.5 per cent). However, improved survival associated with management by a multidisciplinary team at a joint clinic remained significant (RR 0.73, p≤0.001) after adjusting for the effect for prescribing platinum chemotherapy.

Platinum chemotherapy

Clinical trials have shown that platinum chemotherapy improves survival, but can it be shown that, by using chemotherapy, or more specifically certain types of chemotherapy, survival is influenced on a population basis?

Again in studies for the Scottish population (Junor *et al.* 1994), the use of platinum chemotherapy, when compared with non-platinum chemotherapy or no chemotherapy at all, has been shown to improve significantly survival after adjustment for prognostic variables along with the volume of residual disease. Patients prescribed platinum, either alone or in combination with another (non-taxane) drug had a 28 per cent reduction in the chance of dying. More recently, the same group has examined two-year survival rates of patients diagnosed in Scotland in 1993, compared with the population diagnosed with ovarian cancer in 1987. When examined by age group, there had been a 13 per cent improvement in two-year survival rates for patients aged 65–74 years and a 7 per cent improvement in two-year survival rates for patients aged over 75 years. The use of platinum chemotherapy had increased from 20 to 53 per cent and from 3.2 to 13.9 per cent for patients aged 65–74 and over 75 years respectively from 1987 to 1993. For patients aged 64–75, the relative risk of dying had dropped from 1 for patients diagnosed in 1987 to 0.63 for patients with exactly the same characteristics diagnosed in 1993 (p≤0.05), but this difference disappeared entirely when platinum was introduced into the survival model indicating that the improved survival was due to increased use of platinum (Junor & Hole 1997).

Guideline management

In 1991, guidelines on the management of ovarian cancer were issued and circulated in England and Wales by the Standing Subcommittee of Cancer of the Standing Medical Advisory Committee (1991). A similar set of guidelines were developed and circulated in Scotland (Clinical Resource and Audit Group 1995).

Based on these guidelines, local guidelines were developed in various areas of the UK. Wolfe *et al.* (1997) have reported on an audit of the use of local guidelines in South East Thames. This prospective audit of 118 incident cases registered in 1991 across seven district health authorities revealed that only 43 per cent of women were appropriately managed according to those criteria defined in the guidelines. Sixty-six per cent of those treated in teaching hospitals, 45 per cent in non-teaching hospitals with oncology support and 28 per cent in non-teaching hospitals were managed appropriately. Using Cox's proportional hazard model, the risk of death was significantly higher for those patients deemed to have been inappropriately treated (RR 1.48 95 per cent CI 1.34–4.78 p≤0.0043). What the study shows is that despite the issuing of guidelines, less than 50 per cent of patients were managed in accordance with them. The fact that more patients in the teaching hospitals were managed according to guidelines may have nothing to do with the issuing of guidelines and may reflect practice which was already carried out prior to the formation of guidelines. Only a study which directly compares practice before and after guideline development will allow the place of guidelines for ovarian cancer management to be assessed.

Conclusions

Where do we go now? If we think we know which features improve survival for women with ovarian cancer, how do we ensure that all women receive treatment in accordance with these proven factors?

References

Advanced Ovarian Cancer Trialists Group (1991). Chemotherapy in advanced ovarian cancer: an overview of randomised clinical trials. *Br Med J* **303**, 884–93.

Clinical Outcome Indicators Working Group (1996). *Survival from selected cancers by health board*. Clinical Outcome Indicators. The Scottish Office.

Clinical Resource and Audit Group (1995). *Management of ovarian cancer: a report from a working group set up by the Clinical Resource and Audit Group*. Chairman Dr Naren Patel.

The Eurocare Study (1995). *Survival of cancer patients in Europe*. IARC 132.

Forman D & Rider L (ed.) (1996). *Cancer in Yorkshire*. Cancer Registry Report, Cancer Statistics 1989–93.

Kehoe S, Powell J, Wilson S & Woodman C (1994). The influence of operating surgeon's specialisation on patient survival in ovarian carcinoma. *Br J Cancer* **70**, 1014–17.

Griffiths C T (1975). Surgical resection of tumour bulk in the primary treatment of ovarian cancer. *Natl Cancer Inst Monogr* **42**, 101–4.

Junor E J & Hole D J (1997). *Ovarian cancer: survival relative to age and the effect of treatment*. Proceedings EWOC5.

Junor E J, Hole D J & Gillis C R (1994). Management of ovarian cancer: referral to a multidisciplinary team matters. *Br J Cancer* **70**, 363–70.

Junor E J, Hole D J & Gillis C R (1996). Location of treatment: impact on survival. In *Ovarian cancer 4* (ed. F Sharp, T Blackett, R Leake & J Berek). Chapman and Hall Medical, London.

Junor E J, Hole D J, McNulty L, Mason M & Young J (1999). Specialist gynaecologists and survival outcome in ovarian cancer: a Scottish national study of 1866 patients. *Br J Obstet Gynaecol* (in press).

McGuire W P, Hoskins WJ, Brady M F *et al.* (1996). Cyclophosphamide and cisplatin compared with paclitaxel and cisplatin in patients with stage III and stage IV ovarian cancer. *N Eng J Med* **334**, 1–6.

Miller B A, Ries L A G, Hanley B F *et al.* (ed.) (1993). *SEER cancer statistics review 1973–1990.* National Cancer Institute NIH 93-2789.

Standing Subcommittee on Cancer of the Standing Medical Advisory Committee (1991). *Management of ovarian cancer. Current clinical practices. Report of a working group.* Chairman Professor JS Scott. Standing Subcommittee on Cancer of the Standing Medical Advisory Committee, Leeds (pp.1–50).

Stuart G, Bertelsen K, Mangioni C *et al.* (1998). Updated analysis shows a highly significant improved overall survival for cisplatin-paclitaxel as first line treatment of advanced ovarian cancer: mature results of the EORTC-GCCG, NOCOVA, NCIC CTG and Scottish Intergroup Trial. *Proceedings ASCO 1998.*

West Midlands Regional Health Authority (1995). *Cancer and health.* Joint Report of the West Midlands Regional Director of Public Health and the West Midlands Regional Cancer Registry. West Midlands Regional Health Authority.

Wolfe C D A, Tilling K & Raju K S (1997). Management and survival of ovarian cancer patients in South East England. *Eur J Cancer* **33**, 1835–40.

Woodman C, Baghdady A, Collins S & Clyma J-A (1997). What changes in the organisation of cancer services will improve the outcome for women with ovarian cancer? *Br J Obstet Gynaecol* **104**, 135–9.

Chapter 10

Commissioning clinical services for ovarian cancer in *The new NHS*: towards evidence-based policy making

Robbie Foy

Introduction

The word 'purchasing', originally in the title of this chapter, has recently been superseded by 'commissioning'. This is reminiscent of George Orwell's political satire, *1984*, wherein the Ministry of Truth continually rewrote history to control the present: one day the people of the totalitarian state, Oceania, were at war with Eastasia and allied to Eurasia; the next they were at war with Eurasia and allied to Eastasia. Such a reorientation has become a frequent event in the health service where, in 1997, the White Paper, *The new NHS*, (Secretary of State for Health 1997) signalled a switch from purchasing and the competition of the internal market to commissioning and co-operation. One day, clinicians are at war with the purchasers; the next, the commissioners are their allies.

Initially, it was thought that the introduction of the internal market would involve negotiations a little like alcohol clinics, with purchasers banging contracts onto tables and recommending compliance. However, purchasers and providers of health care were intrinsically tied to one another; if the viability of one was severely damaged so was the other. Furthermore, contracts, by themselves, could not change the behaviour and patterns of care provided by a complex health service. Therefore, both purchasers and providers had to develop more collaborative ways of working towards, at least in part, mutual aims. If deciding what these aims are is difficult, achieving them is far harder.

In aiming to improve clinical services for women with ovarian cancer, commissioners need to address the following questions:

- why is the *status quo* unacceptable?
- what service models, processes and outcomes should we pursue?
- how can effective collaboration with clinicians develop in the 'new' NHS?
- is evidence-based commissioning feasible?

These questions are considered below.

Why is the *status quo* unacceptable?

Problems in the provision of clinical services for ovarian cancer which demand change – most importantly, variations in access to a high standard of care and outcomes – have previously been highlighted. Survival independently correlated with specialty of initial assessor and operator (Junor *et al.* 1994; Kehoe *et al.* 1994; Woodman *et al.* 1997), effective chemotherapy and referral to multidisciplinary clinics (Junor *et al.* 1994). Yet as many as half of women with ovarian cancer may not be referred to an oncologist (Woodman *et al.* 1997). One prospective audit (Wolfe *et al.* 1997) demonstrated that despite the presence of clinical guidelines over half (57 per cent) of women in one region were managed inappropriately, receiving inadequate diagnostic investigations and treatment.

In Scotland, the Accounts Commission found variable responses between health boards to the dissemination of national guidelines (Clinical Resource and Audit Group 1995; Accounts Commission for Scotland 1997). Patients are frequently not referred to a specialist gynaecologist, nor referred to combined clinics, nor entered into clinical trials. Despite guideline recommendations, local audits do not take place consistently nor are their findings reported routinely to health boards. Therefore, many health boards are not in a position to ensure that patients receive treatment in line with recommended practice.

The wider environment of the NHS is changing too. Rising expectations of patients and their advocates, more systematic approaches to clinical risk management, the need to justify practice based upon the best available evidence and pressures to make optimal use of limited resources all compel us to reassess the way we plan and deliver health care. The Government's declared commitment to equitable access to high-quality care appears to be more than a policy fashion statement, given the response to the Bristol paediatric cardiac surgery incident and the prominence attached to clinical governance in the White Paper (Smith 1998). Clinical governance broadly entails corporate responsibility for ensuring clinical standards. For the first time, trust chief executives will carry personal and ultimate responsibility for assuring the quality of services, just as they are presently accountable for the proper use of resources. Despite this unprecedented scrutiny of standards of health care, clinical governance should entail more positive levers and mechanisms to promote best practice within trusts.

What models of care should commissioners pursue?

How should commissioners of clinical services for ovarian cancer respond? The Calman/Hine 'hub and spoke' model for England and Wales is based upon a pattern of cancer centres handling the most specialist aspects of care, cancer units following protocols for management of the more common cancers and the continuity of primary care (Department of Health 1995). This model sets out to optimise management from screening and early diagnosis to cure or palliative care, based upon a number of guiding principles:

- access to a uniformly high quality of care;
- public and professional education to help early recognition of symptoms of cancer and the availability of national screening programmes;
- informed choices for patients, families and carers about treatment options and outcomes;
- patient-centred development of cancer services;
- effective communication between all sectors involved with cancer services;
- consistent consideration of psychosocial aspects of cancer care;
- cancer registration and careful monitoring of treatment and outcomes.

Moving towards this model poses several challenges for trusts and health authorities, mainly in allocating the right balance of resources between specialist and generalist care and changing the clinical behaviours and referral patterns of hospital clinicians (Kitchener 1997). Trusts will anticipate adverse impacts on their local services and threats to their viability from being left out in the cold with neither cancer centre nor unit status. Local clinicians will have their autonomy and perceived skills challenged amid fears of becoming 'deskilled'.

There is also a risk that commissioners will practise non-evidence-based policy making by becoming preoccupied with throughput quotas at cancer centres and units rather than quality of care. Much research examining the relationship between patient volume and health outcomes is of poor quality and does not adequately adjust for differences in patient case mix (Nuffield Institute for Health 1996). Overall, the best research suggests that there is no relationship between volume and outcome. However, in selected specialties there appear to be improvements in clinical outcomes associated with increased hospital or clinician volume, a trend supported by some studies assessing cancer care (Selby *et al*. 1998). It is clear that women with ovarian cancer should not be managed single-handedly by a gynaecologist who sees about one or two cases a year. It is intuitive that the more cases one treats, the better the outcomes will be. But the additional benefits of increasing throughput appear to diminish rapidly. Perhaps this is because clinicians overcome 'learning curve' effects or their units work to protocols with better facilities, more skilled supporting staff, and good interspecialty links. Furthermore, although driven by economic imperatives, projected savings from amalgamating smaller into larger units may not be realisable because, as hospitals become larger and more difficult to manage, diseconomies of scale start to appear above 600 beds (Nuffield Institute for Health 1996).

The 'hub and spoke' model is hierarchical and therefore inherently suited to highly specialised tertiary services. But structural change cannot, by itself, guarantee universally improved care. The model should involve more than putting a spin on the centralisation of care and the withdrawal of local autonomy; designated cancer units need support and partnerships. Limited evidence from experience of managing different cancers supports the use of networks based across specialist and general hospitals (Selby *et al.* 1998).

Hence, in Scotland, the emphasis will be on developing 'managed clinical networks' (SoDoH 1998). Partly based on Calman/Hine principles, these networks will be organised around specialty or disease groupings and pooling skills and resources across a number of hospitals. However, these networks must be actively managed, and recognise and build upon existing clinical relationships. An ovarian cancer network will need the collaboration of gynaecologists, oncologists and other specialists, including public health physicians, in developing detailed descriptions of services, integrated protocols and pathways. This, ideally, will expose clinicians to peer review and provide a mechanism for updating protocols and practice. The network rather than individual hospitals will become responsible for attaining a critical mass of patient throughput which facilitates good practice, research and audit. Participation is unlikely to be optional. On top of clinical governance, local general practitioners, primary care groups and community health councils will quickly realise and demand action if one of their local gynaecologists is not acting within a network.

The success of Calman/Hine and managed clinical networks will depend critically on what activities are going on within them to ensure the implementation of evidence-based practice. There is still a considerable gap between research knowledge and its incorporation into routine clinical care. Some of this gap is inevitably related to inadequate resources. But a substantial proportion of the gap is attributable to arcane approaches to education and training. Traditional educational methods, such as the distribution of printed educational materials and didactic lectures, have consistently been shown to be ineffective at improving clinical practice (Davis *et al.* 1995; Freemantle *et al.* 1997). The Cochrane Collaboration on Effective Practice and Organisation of Care is reviewing the effectiveness of interventions to support improved professional practice (see Box 10.1).

There is no single 'magic bullet' to ensure evidence is put into practice (Oxman *et al.* 1995). However, the care of patients with ovarian cancer is more likely to improve if clinicians and managers work to identify barriers to evidence-based practice and use a variety of interventions to promote it. The dissemination of guidelines needs to be reinforced by measures such as interactive educational meetings, clinical prompts, and local audit (Nuffield Institute for Health 1994). Curiously, no systematic review has yet addressed the effectiveness of ministerial exhortations to do better or threats to sack clinicians who do not comply with agreed guidelines. Whatever model of cancer care is adopted, it is should be based upon thriving, interlinked medical communities: 'The central theme of medical diffusion studies is that physicians act as communities rather than aggregates of unrelated individuals and that medical behaviour is literally contagious' (Dixon 1990).

Box 10.1 Evidence on the impact of interventions to promote good practice

Consistent effect	• Prompts and reminders
	• Interactive educational meetings
	• Educational outreach visits
	• Combinations of interventions
Variable effect	• Patient interventions (e.g. leaflets)
	• Audit and feedback on performance
	• Local opinion leaders
	• Local consensus processes
Little or no effect	• Didactic education (e.g. lectures)
	• Educational materials (e.g. guidelines)

[*Source:* Bero *et al.* 1998]

Assessing the work of ovarian cancer services

How should commissioners evaluate ovarian cancer care? It has been recommended that commissioners are responsible for ensuring (Accounts Commission for Scotland 1997):

- identification of consultant gynaecologists with experience in the management of ovarian cancer;
- all patients in whom the diagnosis of ovarian cancer is made are referred to an appropriate gynaecologist who can ensure that an adequate resection has been carried out;
- universal access to a combined gynaecology/oncology service which uses appropriate chemotherapy protocols based on guidelines;
- audit of the number of chemotherapy cycles administered per patient together with the number of drugs involved;
- all patients diagnosed as having ovarian cancer are registered with their regional cancer registry;
- the monitoring of one-, three- and five-year survival figures for their cancer population.

Population survival figures are important to commissioners in two respects. First, they assess the impact over the whole district population of a clinical service. An individual unit may have good survival figures, but it is also necessary to assess the impact over the whole population, thereby including patients not referred and managed appropriately. Accurate and comprehensive cancer registries are vital in this respect. Second, survival statistics should provoke questions. For example, is survival poorer in one district than in another because of wider public health problems, more advanced disease at presentation, high levels of co-morbidity, poorer access to specialised care or suboptimal referral and clinical management (SoDoH 1998)? It is vital that local survival figures are not hijacked and misused in political debates. They need to be viewed within the context of peer-reviewed audit using explicit, measurable standards to assess the appropriateness of care within standardised populations.

Commissioners should encourage audit of entry into clinical trials, not only because they are associated with better outcomes for patients (Stiller 1994), but also in recognition of the need to support high-quality research. However, means of accrediting and rewarding professionals are needed to ensure, for example, that clinicians receive as much credit for enrolling five patients into a multicentre trial as for conducting inconclusive local studies.

Is evidence-based commissioning feasible?

The development of ovarian cancer services requires close collaboration between commissioners and clinicians. However, evidence-based commissioning is difficult in such a fast-changing field (Foy *et al.* 1999). Trusts and health authorities both have to contend with growing clinical demands, limited resources and trying to ensure equal access to new treatments across district boundaries (to prevent 'rationing by postcode'). Commissioners and clinicians will need to work together within the new models envisaged for cancer care to search for and appraise evidence on new interventions and set priorities for funding. This process will need to be multidisciplinary and will inevitably involve reconciling the perspectives of, say, oncologists with clinical expertise and public health physicians with an interest in and experience of assessing new health technologies. This requires tact and toleration on both sides: when negotiations are going badly, both parties may invoke mirror-image claims of underfunding or that they know best how to practise evidence-based medicine.

In April 1999, NHS regional offices became responsible for commissioning specialist services, although health authorities and primary care groups still have a major say in the commissioning of local cancer services (Secretary of State for Health 1997). Nevertheless, there are several problematic issues which need to be addressed, some of which may be ameliorated following implementation of *The new NHS*. These include the following:

- *Information about costs.* At present it is difficult for commissioners to compare the tertiary cancer services provided for their residents with those elsewhere. It is similarly difficult to weigh demands by local cancer specialists for additional resources against other demands. Some benchmarking of specialist cancer hospitals has begun (Richards & Parrott 1996). However, under the White Paper, NHS trusts are required to publish their costs on a consistent basis, and the data published in a national schedule of reference costs so that performance can be compared between trusts.

- *Rewarding good practice and innovation.* At present, inpatient activity is reimbursed at a higher rate than outpatient activity. Therefore, moving interventions to outpatient settings, which may be more convenient for patients and cost-effective, invokes financial penalties for NHS trusts. This 'catch 22' situation could be remedied if new approaches to measuring efficiency are developed, as promised in *The new NHS*.

- *Agreeing criteria to judge the effectiveness of new interventions.* Evidence on new developments is frequently limited despite intense pressure to introduce them. Clinicians and commissioners need to decide on common criteria about what constitutes satisfactory evidence of effectiveness before detailed negotiations begin. Otherwise, both parties might end up talking at cross-purposes. Disagreements might otherwise centre on different values placed on certain trial outcomes (e.g. tumour response rates) or the clinical significance of improvements in mortality or morbidity. Some of these differences would also be easier to resolve if more new drug trials incorporated relevant health and economic outcomes. New agents indicated primarily for palliation might fail to receive funding if trials do not incorporate validated quality of life measurements.

- *Data on cost-effectiveness.* Unfortunately, many studies evaluating new interventions fail to incorporate prospective economic evaluations (Jefferson 1998). Yet, such information is vital in making decisions about how to allocate scant resources. In the absence of sound economic analyses, the use of local data often provides a more timely and relevant basis on which to estimate cost-effectiveness (Mason *et al.* 1993) and inform resource allocation.

- *Promoting equity.* Even when commissioners set out to use explicit and systematic methods of priority setting, their judgement about where to draw the line for funding interventions may still be influenced by resource constraints and pressure from local clinicians (Foy *et al.* 1999). This may partly contribute to unequal access to new treatments, such as paclitaxel in advanced ovarian cancer. The advent of clinical governance, effective use of clinical networks and national guidance may also promote more consistent prescribing between districts. The planned National Institute for Clinical Excellence will be responsible for producing and disseminating clinical guidelines. National service frameworks will set out the patterns and levels of service which should be provided for patients with certain conditions. There is no guarantee that a national centre will be able to generate unambiguous guidance for health technologies because scientific evidence about new technologies is rarely accepted universally, as witnessed by the debate over the use of albumin (Cochrane Injuries Group Albumin Reviewers 1998).

National guidance will need to take account of competing calls on limited resources. As advocates for their patients, clinicians may perceive systematic attempts to set priorities for new cancer drugs as unresponsive to individual patient needs. The NHS already rations health care implicitly using combinations of restricted access to treatment, payment for certain services, waiting lists and, arguably, clinical judgement (New 1998). There are advantages to implicit rationing but it places the burden of individual rationing decisions with doctors and their patients, or with health authorities and trusts. Implicit rationing exacerbates inequalities in access to health care and, arguably, hides rather than highlights the need for additional health care resources. Although it will be inherently difficult, more transparency is needed to help justify how we allocate money within the health service.

Conclusions

Commissioning is not an exact science. Nevertheless, evidence-based commissioning should address three areas: the validity, cost-effectiveness and relevance of biomedical evidence available to support current and new interventions; whether reorganisations of cancer care, through Calman/Hine or managed clinical networks, do reduce variations in care and improve outcomes; and the methods used locally to ensure implementation of evidence-based practice.

Enormous scope exists to improve the care of patients with ovarian cancer. This can be predominantly driven by clinicians but, if clinicians do not take the lead in tackling deficiencies in service provision, clinical governance and chief executives personally responsible for the quality of care will be watchfully behind, perhaps with the keys to Room 101 in their hands. Open, collaborative working will be essential to develop ovarian cancer and other services. This will entail working within and between specialities and work with local commissioners of health care. It will also mean making sacrifices and developing uncomfortable relationships. But some creative tension might be more productive than cosy compromise. In making claims for additional resources, clinicians must share the onus in providing some evidence on cost-effectiveness. However, there is a major need for trials of new interventions, especially of cancer treatments, to incorporate concurrent economic analyses and validated measures of quality of life as well as data on survival. National guidance may help decision making, especially in promoting a fairer distribution of resources, but it remains to be seen whether such guidance can be used as a basis for more open priority setting.

Acknowledgements

I am grateful to Dr Elizabeth Rous and other colleagues for their advice, although the views expressed in this chapter are my own.

References

Accounts Commission for Scotland (1997). *Fighting the silent killer. Optimising the management of ovarian cancer in Scotland.* Accounts Commission for Scotland, Edinburgh.

Bero L A, Grilli R, Grimshaw J M, Harvey E, Oxman A D & Thomson M A (on behalf of the Clinical Resource and Audit Group) (1995). *Management of ovarian cancer.* HMSO, London.

Cochrane Effective Practice and Organisation of Care Review Group (1998). Closing the gap between research and practice: an overview of systematic interventions to promote the implementation of research findings. *BMJ* **317**, 465–8.

Cochrane Injuries Group Albumin Reviewers (1998). Human albumin administration in critically ill patients: systematic review of randomised controlled trials. *BMJ* **317**, 235–40.

Davis D A *et al.* (1995). Changing physician performance: a systematic review of the effect of continuing medical education strategies. *JAMA* **274**, 700–5.

Department of Health (1995). *A policy framework for commissioning cancer services.* HM Stationery Office, London, p.18.

Dixon A (1990). The evolution of clinical policies. *Medical Care* **28**, 201–20.

Foy R, So J, Rous E & Scarffe H (1999). Commissioner and specialist perspectives of prioritising new cancer drugs: impact of the evidence threshold. *BMJ* **318**, 456–9.

Freemantle N, Harvey E L, Wolf F, Grimshaw J M, Grilli R & Bero L A (1997). *Printed educational materials to improve the behaviour of health care professionals and patient outcomes.* Collaboration on Effective Professional Practice Module of The Cochrane Database of Systematic Reviews.

Jefferson T (1998). Concurrent economic evaluations are rare but should be standard practice. *BMJ* **317**, 915–16.

Junor E J, Hole D J & Gillis C R (1994). Management of ovarian cancer: referral to a multidisciplinary team matters. *Br J Cancer* **70**, 363–70.

Kehoe S, Powell J, Wilson S & Woodman C (1994). The influence of the operating surgeon's specialisation on patient survival in ovarian carcinoma. *Br J Cancer* **70**, 1014–17.

Kitchener H (1997). Gynaecological cancer services: time for change. *Br J Obstet Gynaecol* **104**, 123–6.

Mason J, Drummond M & Torrance G (1993). Some guidelines on the use of cost-effectiveness league tables. *BMJ* **306**, 570–2.

New B (on behalf of the Rationing Agenda Group) (1998). The rationing agenda in the NHS. *BMJ* **312**, 1593–601.

Nuffield Institute for Health (1994). *Implementing clinical practice guidelines*. Effective Health Care, University of Leeds, Leeds.

Nuffield Institute for Health, NHS Centre for Reviews and Dissemination (1996). *Hospital volume and health care outcomes, costs and patient access*. Effective Health Care, University of York, York.

Oxman A D, Thomson M A, Davis D A & Haynes R B (1995). No magic bullets: a systematic review of 102 trials of interventions to help health care professionals deliver services more effectively or efficiently. *Can Med Assoc J* **153**, 1423–31.

Richards MA & Parrott (on behalf of the 12 participating centres) (1996). Tertiary cancer services in Britain: benchmarking study of activity and facilities at 12 specialist centres. *BMJ* **313**, 347–9.

Secretary of State for Health (1997). *The new NHS*. Stationery Office, London (Cm 3807).

Selby P, Gillis C & Haward R (1996). Benefits from specialised cancer care. *Lancet* **348**, 313–18.

Smith R (1998). All changed, changed utterly. *BMJ* **316**, 1917–18.

SoDoH (1998). *Acute services review report*. SoDoH.

Stiller C A (1994). Centralised treatment, entry to trials and survival. *Br J Cancer* **70**, 352–62.

Wolfe C D A, Tilling K & Raju K S (1997). Management and survival of ovarian cancer patients in South East England. *Eur J Cancer* **33**(11), 1835–40.

Woodman C, Baghdady A, Collins S & Clyma J-A (1997). What changes in the organisation of cancer services will improve the outcome for women with ovarian cancer? *Br J Obstet Gynaecol* **104**, 135–9.

Index